Fungal Infection

DIAGNOSIS
AND MANAGEMENT

Fungal Infection

DIAGNOSIS
AND MANAGEMENT

Malcolm D. Richardson

BSc, PhD, CBiol, MIBiol, MRCPath
Consultant Clinical Scientist in Mycology
Regional Mycology Reference Laboratory
Department of Dermatology
University of Glasgow and Western Infirmary
Glasgow

David W. Warnock

BSc, PhD, MRCPath
Consultant Clinical Scientist in Mycology
PHLS Mycology Reference Laboratory
Public Health Laboratory, Bristol

Presented as a service to medicine
with the compliments of Vestar

b

Blackwell
Science

First published 1993
Reprinted 1994 (five times)

Set by Excel Typesetters Company,
Hong Kong
Printed and bound in Great Britain by
Biddles Ltd, Guildford and King's Lynn

DISTRIBUTORS
Marston Book Services Ltd
PO Box 87
Oxford OX2 ODT
(*Orders*: Tel: 01865 791155
     Fax: 01865 791927
     Telex: 837515)

USA
Blackwell Science, Inc.
238 Main Street
Cambridge, MA 02142
(*Orders*: Tel: 800 759-6102
     617 876-7000)

Canada
Times Mirror Professional Publishing, Ltd
130 Flaska Drive
Markham, Ontario L6G 1B8
(*Orders*: Tel: 800 268-4178
     416 470-6739)

Australia
Blackwell Science Pty Ltd
54 University Street
Carlton, Victoria 3053
(*Orders*: Tel: 03 347-5552)

A catalogue record for this title
is available from the British Library

ISBN 0-632-03514-5

Library of Congress
Cataloging in Publication Data

Richardson, M.D.
    Fungal Infection: diagnosis and
    management/
    Malcolm D. Richardson, David W.
    Warnock.
         p.   cm.
    Includes bibliographical references
    and index.
    ISBN 0-632-03514-5
    1. Mycoses.   I. Warnock, D.W.
    II. Title.
    [DNLM: 1. Mycoses—diagnosis.
    2. Mycoses—therapy. WC 450 R524f
      1993]
    RC117.R47 1993
    616.9'69—dc20

Contents

Preface

Fungal infections are assuming a greater importance, largely because of their increasing incidence among transplant patients and other immunocompromised individuals, including those with AIDS. As a result, clinicians and microbiologists alike need to be familiar with the clinical presentation and methods for the diagnosis of these infections, as well as the current treatment choices.

In this book we have attempted to provide a succinct account of the clinical manifestations, laboratory diagnosis and management of fungal infections found in European, American and Australasian practice. The book covers problems encountered both in hospitals and general practice, and is designed to permit clinicians to make the best use of the various laboratory investigations available. Emphasis is placed on clinical presentation, specimen collection, interpretation of laboratory findings, and choice of treatment regimen. In general, the length of the chapters reflects the frequency or the importance of the clinical problems, or both.

We have designed this book to facilitate rapid information retrieval. Our reading list of established literature has been carefully selected to permit efficient access to specific aspects of fungal infections and has been annotated to guide the reader.

We hope this book will be of interest to medical students, junior hospital medical staff, hospital specialists and general practitioners. In particular it should appeal to microbiologists, infectious disease specialists, dermatologists, haematologists, genitourinary medicine specialists, oncologists and intensive-care staff.

M.D.R., D.W.W.

Acknowledgements

We would like to thank the staff of the mycology laboratories in Glasgow and Bristol whose support and help during the various stages of preparation of this book has been invaluable. Especial thanks are due to our wives and families for their tolerance and encouragement.

M.D.R., D.W.W.

1   Introduction

The nature of fungi

Living organisms are now divided up among no fewer than
five Kingdoms, one of which is the Kingdom Fungi. This
Kingdom comprises a diverse group of eukaryotic organisms
that have definite cell walls and are devoid of chlorophyll.
Thus, all fungi must lead a heterotrophic existence in nature
as parasites or saprobes, dependent on living or dead organic
matter for their nutrients.

The classification and identification of fungi is based on
their appearance, rather than on the nutritional and bio-
chemical differences that are of such importance in bacterial
classification. In most fungi, the vegetative phase consists of
filaments or hyphae, with numerous lateral branches, which
together form the mycelium. While the hyphae of the more
primitive fungi remain aseptate (without cross-walls), those
of the more advanced groups are septate, that is partitioned
by more or less frequent cross-walls. Under certain conditions, additional septa may be laid down in the hyphae,
which then fragment into chains of resting spores, termed
arthrospores.

In one large group of fungi, termed the yeasts, the organism consists of separate round, oval or elongated cells that
propagate by budding out similar cells from their surface.
Under certain conditions the cells remain attached, forming
a chain of elongated cells or pseudomycelium. Many fungi,
including some of medical importance, can exist in a mycelial
or a yeast form depending on the environmental conditions.

The classification of fungi is based on the method of
sexual reproduction. However, one group (termed the Fungi
Imperfecti) is an artificial one and contains all the fungi
for which no method of sexual reproduction has been
discovered. Members of this group often produce great
numbers of asexual spores (termed conidia) which are
often formed on specialized aerial structures (termed conidiophores). The shape and size of the spores, and the
arrangement of the spore-bearing structures, are of major
importance in identification.

Should both the sexual (teleomorph) and asexual (anamorph) stage of a given fungus be known, it is almost certain

that different names will have been applied to them. Both these names are valid under the International Code of Botanical Nomenclature, but that of the teliomorph should take precedence over that of the anamorph. In practice, however, it is common to refer to organisms of medical importance by their asexual designations (such as *Trichophyton mentagrophytes*) because the anamorphic form is isolated from clinical specimens, rather than their teleomorphic designation (*Arthroderma benhamiae*) because the sexual form is only obtained in culture.

1.2   Fungi as human pathogens

Among the 50 000 to 250 000 species of fungi that have been described, fewer than 200 have been associated with human disease. In general these organisms are free-living in nature and are in no way dependent on humans (or animals) for their survival. With few exceptions, fungal infections of humans originate from an exogenous source in the environment and are acquired through inhalation, ingestion or traumatic implantation.

A handful of fungi are capable of causing significant disease in otherwise normal individuals. Many more are only able to produce disease under unusual circumstances, mostly involving host debilitation. However, as a result of the numerous developments in modern medicine, these hitherto innocuous organisms have gained increasing prominence as aetiological agents of disease. Any fungus capable of growing at the temperature of the host (37°C) and surviving in a lowered oxidation–reduction state (a situation found in damaged tissue) must now be regarded as a potential human pathogen.

Fungal infections can be classified into a number of broad groups according to the initial site of infection. Grouping the diseases in this manner brings out clearly the degree of parasitic adaptation of the different groups of fungi and the way in which the site affected is related to the route by which the fungus enters the host.

1.2.1
The superficial mycoses

These are infections limited to the outermost layers of the skin, the nails and hair, and the mucous membranes. The principal infections in this group are the dermatophytoses and superficial forms of candidosis. Many of these infections are mild and readily diagnosed, and respond well to treatment.

The dermatophytes are limited to the keratinized tissues

of the epidermis, hair and nail. Most are unable to survive as free-living saprobes in competition with other keratinophilic organisms in the environment and thus are dependent on passage from host to host for their survival. These obligate pathogens seem to have evolved from unspecialized saprobic forms. In the process, most are now no longer capable of sexual reproduction and some are even incapable of asexual reproduction. In general, these organisms have become well adapted to humans, evoking little or no inflammatory reaction from the host.

The aetiological agents of candidosis, like the dermatophytes, are entirely dependent on the living host for their survival, but differ from them in the manner by which this is achieved. These organisms, of which *Candida albicans* is the most important, are normal commensals of the human digestive tract, including the mouth. Acquisition of these organisms from another host seldom results in overt disease, but rather results in the setting-up of a commensal relationship with the new host. These organisms do not produce disease unless some change in the circumstances of the host lowers its natural defences. In this situation, endogenous infection from the host's own reservoir of the organism may result in mucosal, cutaneous or deep-seated infection. In recent years, disseminated candidosis has emerged as a relatively common, life-threatening illness in debilitated or immunosuppressed patients.

1.2.2
The subcutaneous mycoses

These are infections involving the dermis, subcutaneous tissues and bone. These infections are usually acquired as a result of the traumatic implantation of organisms that grow as saprobes in soil and decomposing vegetation. These infections are most frequently encountered among the rural populations of the tropical and subtropical regions of the world, where individuals go barefoot and wear the minimum of clothing. The disease may remain localized at the site of implantation or spread to adjacent tissue. More widespread dissemination of the infection, through the blood or lymphatics, is uncommon and usually only occurs if the host is in some way debilitated.

1.2.3
The systemic mycoses

These are infections that usually originate in the lungs, but may spread to many other organs. These infections are most commonly acquired as a result of inhaling spores of organisms that grow as saprobes in soil or decomposing organic matter, or as pathogens on plants.

The organisms that cause systemic fungal infection can be divided into two distinct groups: the true pathogens and the opportunists. The first of these groups consists of a handful of organisms, such as *Histoplasma capsulatum* and *Coccidioides immitis*, that are able to invade and develop in the tissues of a normal host with no recognizable predisposition. Often these organisms possess unique morphological features that appear to contribute to their survival within the host. The second group, the opportunists, consists of less virulent and less well adapted organisms, such as *Aspergillus fumigatus*, that are only able to invade the tissues of a debilitated or immunosuppressed host.

In most cases, infections with true pathogenic fungi are asymptomatic or mild and of short duration. Many cases occur in regions endemic for the fungus and follow inhalation of spores that have been released into the environment. Individuals who recover from these infections enjoy marked and lasting resistance to reinfection, while the few patients with chronic or residual disease develop a granulomatous response.

In addition to their well-recognized manifestations in normal individuals, infections with true pathogenic fungi have emerged as significant diseases in immunosuppressed individuals. Histoplasmosis and coccidioidomycosis, for instance, have been recognized as two of the defining conditions for the acquired immunodeficiency syndrome (AIDS). In debilitated or immunocompromised patients, infections with true pathogenic fungi are often life-threatening and unresponsive to antifungal treatment, or relapse following treatment resulting in death.

Opportunistic fungal infections occur in individuals who are debilitated or immunosuppressed as a result of an underlying disease or their treatment. In most cases, infection results in significant disease. Resolution of the infection does not confer protection, and reinfection or reactivation may occur if host resistance is again lowered. Many of the organisms involved are ubiquitous saprobes, found in the soil, on decomposing organic matter and in the air. Although new species of fungi are regularly being identified as causes of disease in immunosuppressed humans, four diseases still account for most reported infections: aspergillosis, candidosis, cryptococcosis and mucormycosis (zygomycosis).

Many of the systemic fungal infections of humans have a restricted geographical distribution, being limited to regions where the causal organisms occur in nature. For instance,

Coccidioides immitis only occurs in alkaline soils in certain semi-arid parts of southwestern North America, and similar regions in Central and South America, where there are hot summers and few cold periods in winter. Most cases of human coccidioidomycosis are acquired in these regions. On the other hand, *Cryptococcus neoformans* is found wherever there are pigeon droppings, and cases of cryptococcosis occur throughout the world.

In contrast to the restricted geographical distribution of most of the true pathogenic fungi, the spores of many opportunistic fungi are ubiquitous in the environment and often reach high concentrations in hospital air. Nosocomial (hospital-acquired) outbreaks of aspergillosis and other infections have become associated with hospital construction or renovation work in or near units in which immuno-suppressed patients are housed. These outbreaks have high-lighted the need for efficient ventilation with filtered air in such units.

1.3
The changing pattern of fungal infection

Over the past few years, improvements in the management of debilitated medical and surgical patients have led to an unwelcome increase in the number of life-threatening infections due to true pathogenic and opportunistic fungi. These infections are being seen in ever-increasing numbers among cancer patients, transplant recipients and patients receiving broad-spectrum antibiotics or parenteral nutrition. Fungal infection is also becoming more common among other groups of debilitated or seriously ill patients, such as drug addicts and patients with AIDS. Estimates of the incidence of these infections are thought to be quite conservative in comparison with their true magnitude, because many fungal infections go undiagnosed.

In addition to the rise in opportunistic fungal infec-tions due to such well-recognized organisms as *Aspergillus fumigatus* and *Candida albicans*, an ever-increasing number of fungi, hitherto regarded as harmless saprobes, are being reported as the cause of serious or lethal infection in immunosuppressed individuals. For instance, *Trichosporon beigelii*, the aetiological agent of the mild dermatological condition white piedra, is now well documented as a cause of lethal disseminated infection in leukaemic patients and bone marrow transplant (BMT) recipients. The emergence of this organism as a significant pathogen has important implica-tions for diagnosis and management, because the clinical presentation can mimic candidosis but the organism is often resistant to the drug (amphotericin) used to treat that infection. The saprobic soil mould *Pseudallescheria boydii* is another organism that can cause life-threatening infection that mimics a more common condition, aspergillosis. It, too, is often resistant to amphotericin, the drug of choice for aspergillus infection.

Implications for diagnosis and management

The dramatic increase in the number and range of different fungal infections now being reported has been due to a combination of improved recognition and an increasing population of susceptible patients. This rise in prevalence has resulted in an increased awareness of the need for improved methods of diagnosis and for new methods of management. As with other microbial infections, the diagnosis of fungal disease is based upon a combination of clinical observation and laboratory investigation.

Laboratory methods for the diagnosis of fungal infection continue to be updated, but depend for the most part on culture of the fungus, on its detection in clinical material by direct microscopic examination, and on the detection of antibodies using a range of serological procedures. Now that an increasing number of common culture contaminants (and other less usual environmental organisms) are occurring as occasional opportunistic pathogens, it is more important than ever that medical microbiologists should be able to recognize these organisms, at least to genus level. The application of molecular biological techniques to the identification of fungi is attracting attention, and while practical procedures have been developed for distinguishing strains of particular organisms, it is doubtful whether these methods can supplant the traditional morphological approach to mould identification.

Monoclonal antibodies to structural components of the major fungal pathogens of humans are now being produced. These reagents have the potential to form the basis for new tests for identification of organisms. Their introduction has stimulated significant developments in the diagnosis of fungal infection, by enabling improved tests for the detection of circulating fungal antigens in immunosuppressed patients to be devised. Monoclonal-based latex particle agglutination (LPA) and enzyme-linked immunoadsorbent assay (ELISA) tests have now been marketed for the diagnosis of deep candidosis and aspergillosis, as well as for cryptococcosis.

The increased prevalence of life-threatening fungal infection has stimulated interest in the development of new antifungal drugs. New compounds, such as the triazoles and the allylamines, have been introduced and new formulations of older compounds, such as liposomal amphotericin, have appeared. These developments have improved the treatment of many forms of fungal infection, but problems remain. There are still important infections, such as mucormycosis, for which no reliable treatment has been developed. Then again, many strains of the unusual organisms, such as *Candida krusei* and *Trichosporon beigelii*, that are now being isolated from debilitated patients, are insensitive to current antifungal compounds.

2 Laboratory Diagnosis of Fungal Infection

2.1 **Introduction**

As with other microbial infections, the diagnosis of fungal infections depends upon a combination of clinical observation and laboratory investigation. Superficial fungal infections often produce characteristic lesions which suggest a fungal diagnosis, but it is not unusual to find that the appearance of lesions has been modified and rendered atypical by previous treatment. In most situations where deep fungal infection is entertained as a diagnosis, the clinical presentation is nonspecific and can be caused by a wide range of infections, underlying illness or complications of treatment.

Laboratory tests can help in establishing or confirming the diagnosis of a fungal infection, in providing objective assessments of response to treatment and in monitoring resolution of the infection. The successful laboratory diagnosis of fungal infection depends in major part on the collection of appropriate clinical specimens for investigation. It is also dependent on the selection of appropriate microbiological test procedures. These differ from mycosis to mycosis, and depend on the site of infection as well as the presenting symptoms and clinical signs. Interpretation of the results can sometimes be made with confidence, but at times the findings can be unhelpful or even misleading. It is in these situations that close liaison between the clinician and the laboratory is particularly important.

2.2 **Collection of specimens**

To establish or confirm the diagnosis of suspected fungal infection, it is essential for the clinician to provide the laboratory with adequate specimens for investigation. Inappropriate collection, storage or processing of specimens can result in a missed diagnosis. Moreover, to ensure that the most appropriate laboratory tests are performed, it is essential for the clinician to indicate that a fungal infection is suspected and to provide sufficient background information.

In addition to specifying the source of the specimen and its time of collection, it is important to provide information on any underlying illness, recent travel or previous residence abroad, any animal contacts and the patient's occupation. This information will help the laboratory to anticipate which fungal pathogens are most liable to be involved and permit the selection of the most appropriate test procedures. In addition, the laboratory *must* be informed if there are particular risks associated with the handling of the specimen, for instance if the patient has hepatitis or is human immunodeficiency virus (HIV)-positive.

With the exception of skin, hair and nails, specimens for mycological examination should be collected into and transported to the laboratory in sterile containers appropriate to the type of material being investigated. All specimen containers must be clearly labelled.

2.2.1
Skin, nails and hair

It is often helpful to clean cutaneous and scalp lesions (and sometimes nails) with 70% alcohol prior to sampling as this will improve the chances of detecting fungus on microscopic examination, as well as reducing the likelihood of bacterial contamination of cultures. Prior cleaning is essential if ointments, creams or powders have been applied to the lesion.

Skin, nail and hair specimens should be collected into folded squares of black paper (about 10 cm × 10 cm). The use of paper permits the specimen to dry out, which helps to reduce bacterial contamination and also provides a convenient means of storing specimens for long periods (12 months or longer).

Material should be collected from cutaneous lesions by scraping outwards from the margin of the lesion with the edge of a glass microscope slide or a blunt scalpel. If there is minimal scaling, as often occurs with lesions of the glabrous skin, it is helpful to use clear adhesive tape to remove material for examination. The Sellotape strip should be pressed against the lesion, peeled off and placed, adhesive-side-down, on a clean glass microscope slide for transportation to the laboratory.

Specimens from the scalp should include hair roots, the contents of plugged follicles, and skin scales. Hairs should be plucked from the scalp with forceps. Cut hairs without roots are unsuitable for mycological investigation because the infection is usually confined near or below the surface of the scalp.

It is often helpful to use a Wood's light to select infected hairs for laboratory investigation. This portable source of long-wave ultraviolet light can be used to detect the green fluorescence of hair which is a feature of some forms of dermatophyte scalp infection. It is particularly useful for detection of inconspicuous scalp lesions.

Another technique which is useful for collection of adequate material from patients with inconspicuous scalp lesions is hairbrush sampling. The scalp is brushed with a plastic hairbrush or scalp massage pad which is then pressed into the surface of an agar plate. The brushes or pads can be sterilized in 1% chlorhexidine for 1 h, rinsed in sterile water and dried before being reused.

Nail specimens should be taken from any discoloured, dystrophic or brittle parts of the nail. Specimens should be cut as far back as possible from the edge of the nail and should include the full thickness of the nail because some fungi are confined to the lower parts. If the nail is thickened, scrapings can also be taken from beneath it.

2.2.2
Mouth and
vagina

Although scrapings from oral lesions are better than swabs for diagnosis of oral infections, the latter are more frequently used, mainly because they are more convenient for transporting material to the laboratory. Swabs should either be moistened with sterile water or saline prior to taking the sample, or sent to the laboratory in transport medium.

For vaginal infections, swabs should be taken from discharge in the vagina and from the lateral vaginal wall. Swabs should be sent to the laboratory in transport medium.

2.2.3
Ear

Scrapings of material from the ear canal are to be preferred, although swabs can also be used.

2.2.4
Ocular
specimens

Material from patients with suspected fungal infection of the cornea (keratomycosis) should be collected by scraping the ulcer with a sterile platinum spatula. The entire base of the ulcer, as well as the edges, should be scraped. As the amount of material obtained may be very small, it is best transferred directly to agar plates for culture and to a glass slide for microscopic examination. The plates should be marked to indicate where the inoculum has been applied before being transported to the laboratory. Swabs are not suitable for sampling corneal lesions.

In patients with suspected fungal endophthalmitis, vitreous humour should be collected using a pars plana (closed) vitrectomy. Vitreous humour specimens that have been diluted by the irrigating solution should be concentrated by centrifugation before being examined in the laboratory.

2.2.5
Blood

Blood culture should be performed in all cases of suspected deep fungal infection. However, unless specialized techniques or media are used, clinicians should not expect blood cultures taken for isolation of bacteria to detect fungi other than *Candida* species or *Trichosporon* species. Culture of arterial blood should be considered if venous blood cultures are unsuccessful in a patient with suspected deep mycosis.

The most sensitive method for isolation of a wide range of fungal pathogens (including *Cryptococcus neoformans* and *Histoplasma capsulatum*) from blood is the lysis centrifugation technique (DuPont Isolator System). If *Candida* species are being sought, both the radiometric and nonradiometric Bactec Systems are suitable. Both are superior to culture in vented biphasic media or broth.

2.2.6
Cerebrospinal fluid

Cerebrospinal fluid (CSF) specimens (3–5 ml) should be collected by lumbar puncture. Samples can be centrifuged and the supernatant used for serological tests. The sediment can be cultured, but is also useful for microscopic examination.

2.2.7
Urine

In non-catheterized patients, midstream specimens of urine are adequate for mycological investigation, provided care is taken to ensure that vaginal or perineal infection does not lead to contamination. In infants, suprapubic aspiration is the best method of urine collection. High counts of *Candida* species are often encountered in urine cultures from patients with a long-term indwelling catheter. Such counts usually indicate nothing more than colonization of the lower urinary tract or catheter.

Patients with blastomycosis or cryptococcosis may have prostatic infection, making postprostatic massage urine specimens important to collect. The specimen should be centrifuged and the sediment cultured. Other disseminated infections that can be diagnosed on the basis of a positive urine culture include coccidioidomycosis and histoplasmosis.

2.2.8
Other fluids

Chest, abdominal and joint fluids, whether aspirated or drained, should be collected into sterile containers containing a small amount of 1:1000 sterile heparin to prevent clotting. The specimens should be centrifuged and the sediment cultured. Drain fluid from patients on continuous peritoneal dialysis should be collected into a sterile container without heparin.

2.2.9
Lower
respiratory
tract specimens

Sputum specimens should be collected in the morning, soon after awakening, into a sterile container. If possible, the mouth should be rinsed with water before collecting the specimen. If the patient does not have a productive cough, a sputum sample may be induced by introducing nebulized saline into the bronchial tree. Twenty-four-hour collections of sputum are not suitable for mycological investigation.

If possible, sputum specimens should be processed within 2 h of collection. If delay in processing is unavoidable, specimens must be stored at 4°C.

More invasive sampling methods are often needed to obtain lower respiratory tract specimens from immuno-suppressed patients. Percutaneous methods are seldom used now, because of their low rate of success and high rate of complications. Bronchoalveolar lavage, carried out with a fibre-optic bronchoscope, provides useful specimens for microscopic examination and culture.

2.2.10
Pus

The use of swabs to collect material from draining abscesses or ulcers is not recommended. If a swab must be used for sampling, then material should be taken from as deep as possible within the lesion. Pus from undrained subcutaneous abscesses or sinus tracts should be collected with a sterile needle and syringe. If any grains are visible in the pus (as in mycetoma), these must be collected. In mycetoma, if the crusts at the opening of sinus tracts are lifted, grains can often be found in the pus underneath.

2.2.11
Bone marow

These specimens are useful for making the diagnosis in a number of deep fungal infections, including histoplasmosis, cryptococcosis and paracoccidioidomycosis. About 3–5 ml aspirated material should be collected in a sterile container with 0.5 ml of sterile 1 : 1000 heparin.

2.2.12
Tissue

Tissue specimens should be placed in sterile saline and *not* in formalin. If possible, material should be obtained from both the middle and the edge of lesions. Small cutaneous, subcutaneous or mucosal lesions can often be excised completely.

2.3

Specimens for serological tests

Serological tests for fungal pathogens are often more helpful if paired or sequential specimens of serum, urine or CSF are collected.

Blood, CSF and other biological fluids for serological

testing should be collected into glass or plastic tubes without anticoagulants; 5-10 ml is usually sufficient.

2.4 **Specimens for antifungal drug level determinations**

The concentrations in blood of antifungal drugs are measured for two principal reasons: to ensure that adequate drug concentrations are attained and to ensure that concentrations that could cause unpleasant or even harmful side effects are avoided.

Blood and other biological fluids should be collected into glass or plastic tubes without anticoagulants; 5-10 ml is usually sufficient. Care should be taken to ensure that specimens are taken at the most appropriate times: samples should be collected just before a dose is due and/or around the expected time of peak serum concentrations (see Chapter 3).

2.5 **Transport of specimens**

Apart from specimens from cases of suspected dermatophytosis which can often be stored for weeks or even months before processing, specimens for mycological investigation must be processed as soon as possible after collection. Delay may result in the death of fastidious organisms, in overgrowth of contaminants, and/or multiplication in the number of organisms present.

Specimens mailed to laboratories must be packaged and labelled according to the guidelines laid down for the transport of biological material by the relevant postal authorities. Metal canisters are now recommended for packaging of certain hazardous materials, such as specimens from HIV-positive individuals. Plastic Petri dishes are unsuitable for sending through the mail. The specimen container or culture should be sealed within a plastic bag before packaging, so that any breakage and subsequent spillage is contained. The sender's name should be clearly marked on the outside of the package so that he or she may be contacted for instructions should a problem arise.

2.6 **Interpretation of laboratory test results**

Interpretation of the results of laboratory tests can sometimes be made with confidence, but at times the findings may be unhelpful or even misleading. The investigations available include microscopic examination, culture and serological tests. The choice of appropriate tests differs from mycosis to mycosis, and depends on the site of infection as well as the presenting symptoms and clinical signs. It must always be appreciated that every laboratory test has its limitations, and that negative results can be obtained which may lead to unjustified exclusion of a mycological diagnosis.

2.6.1
Direct
microscopic
examination

The direct microscopic examination of clinical material is one of the simpler and most helpful procedures for the laboratory diagnosis of fungal infection. Various methods can be used: unstained wet-mount preparations may be examined by light-field, dark-field or phase-contrast illumination; or dried smears can be stained and examined.

Direct microscopic examination is most useful in the diagnosis of superficial and subcutaneous fungal infections. Recognition of fungal elements in skin scrapings, hair or nail specimens can provide a reliable indication of the mycosis involved, whether it be dermatophytosis, candidosis or pityriasis versicolor. In certain situations, direct microscopic examination of fluids or other clinical material can establish the diagnosis of a deep mycosis. Instances include the detection of encapsulated *Cryptococcus neoformans* cells in CSF, or *Histoplasma capsulatum* cells in peripheral blood smears. More often, however, only a tentative diagnosis of deep fungal infection can be made on the basis of microscopic examination. Nevertheless, this is often sufficient to allow the instigation of antifungal treatment pending the outcome of other investigations.

2.6.2
Culture

With few exceptions the isolation of pathogenic fungi from clinical material is not difficult. Should the isolate be identified as an unequivocal pathogen, such as *Trichophyton rubrum* or *Cryptococcus neoformans*, then the diagnosis is established. If, however, an opportunistic pathogen such as *Aspergillus fumigatus* or *Candida albicans* is recovered, then its isolation may have no clinical relevance unless there is additional evidence of infection. Isolation of opportunistic fungal pathogens from sterile sites, such as blood or CSF, often provides reliable evidence of significant infection, but their isolation from material such as pus, sputum or urine must be interpreted with caution. Attention should be given to the amount of fungus isolated and further investigations undertaken.

Many unfamiliar organisms have been reported to cause deep-seated fungal infection in immunosuppressed patients. No isolate should be dismissed as a contaminant without careful consideration of the clinical condition of the patient, the site of isolation, the method of specimen collection, and the amount of organisms recovered.

Although culture often provides the definitive diagnosis of a fungal infection, it also has some limitations. Chief amongst these is failure to recover the organism. This may be due to inadequate specimen collection or delayed transport of specimens. Incorrect isolation procedures or inadequate periods of incubation are other important factors. It is essential for the clinician to inform the laboratory if a particular fungal infection is suspected and provide sufficient information to permit the most appropriate culture procedures to be followed.

The isolation and identification of a mycelial fungus can take several weeks. In such unavoidable instances, the result may become available too late either to help with the diagnosis or with the choice of treatment. Nevertheless, culture should always be attempted so that a definitive diagnosis can be obtained.

2.6.3
Serological tests

The detection of fungal antibodies is sometimes helpful in the diagnosis of subcutaneous and deep-seated fungal infections. Numerous methods are available. For some infections, such as histoplasmosis and coccidioidomycosis, the tests are reliable, but for others the results are seldom more than suggestive or supportive of a fungal diagnosis. It is often more helpful if sequential tests can be performed, so that rising levels of antibodies may be detected.

Tests for the detection of fungal antibodies are least helpful in immunosuppressed patients. In such cases serological tests for the detection of fungal antigens may be more useful. Antigen detection is an established procedure for the diagnosis of cryptococcosis and similar methods are now being introduced for other mycoses, including aspergillosis, candidosis and histoplasmosis. Because of the low concentrations of circulating antigens present in many infected individuals, sensitive test methods are required.

2.6.4
Histopatho-
logical
examination

The demonstration of fungal elements in histological material is one of the most useful procedures for the diagnosis of subcutaneous and deep-seated fungal infections. The ease with which a fungal pathogen can be recognized in tissue is dependent in part on its abundance, but also on the distinctiveness of its appearance. Although there are a number of special stains for detecting and highlighting fungal cells, specific identification of organisms may be difficult. The detection of nonpigmented, branching, septate mycelium can be indicative of aspergillus infection, but it is also characteristic of a number of less common organisms. Likewise, the detection of small, budding cells in clinical material seldom permits a specific diagnosis. Tissue-form cells of *Histoplasma capsulatum* and *Blastomyces dermatitidis*, for instance, can appear similar and may be confused with nonencapsulated *Cryptococcus neoformans* cells. Immunofluorescence and other immunochemical staining procedures sometimes permit the specific identification of fungal elements in histological sections.

3   Antifungal Drugs

3.1   Introduction

In comparison with the number of antibacterial drugs available, there are far fewer antifungal compounds. Even so the number of antifungal drugs is increasing all the time. There are three major families of compounds: the polyenes, the azoles and the allylamines. In addition there is a miscellaneous group of compounds, such as griseofulvin, which do not belong to one of the major families. This is not a static picture as there are new groups of compounds under development.

This chapter reviews the principal antifungals in current use for superficial, subcutaneous and deep-seated fungal infections.

3.2   Amphotericin

Amphotericin is a macrocyclic polyene antibiotic derived from *Streptomyces nodosus*. It remains the drug of choice for many forms of deep fungal infection.

3.2.1 Mechanism of action

Amphotericin binds to ergosterol, the principal sterol in the membrane of susceptible fungal cells, causing impairment of membrane barrier function, loss of cell constituents, metabolic disruption and cell death. In addition to its membrane permeabilizing effects, the drug can cause oxidative damage to fungal cells.

3.2.2 Spectrum of action

Amphotericin has a broad spectrum of action including *Aspergillus* species, *Blastomyces dermatitidis*, *Candida* species, *Coccidioides immitis*, *Cryptococcus neoformans*, *Histoplasma capsulatum* and *Paracoccidioides brasiliensis*. It is effective in certain forms of mucormycosis, hyalophomycosis and phaeohyphomycosis, but often ineffective in pseudallescheriosis and trichosporonosis.

3.2.3 Acquired resistance

Treatment failure attributable to the development of amphotericin resistance is rare. Resistant strains of *Candida lusitaniae* and *C. tropicalis*, with alterations in the cell membrane including reduced amounts of ergosterol, have been isolated during treatment.

3.2.4 Pharmacokinetics

Amphotericin is not absorbed following mucosal or cutaneous application. Minimal absorption occurs from the gastrointestinal tract. Oral administration of a 3 g dose will produce serum concentrations in the region of 0.1–0.5 mg/l.

Parenteral administration of 1 mg/kg dose of the conventional colloidal dispersion formulation of the drug will produce serum concentrations of 1.0–2.0 mg/l. Administration of a 3 mg/kg dose of liposomal amphotericin (AmBisome) at 24 h intervals will produce serum concentrations in the region of 20 mg/l. The conventional formulation of the drug has an initial serum half-life of about 24–48 h and an elimination half-life of about 2 weeks. The liposomal formulation has an initial serum half-life of about 0.4–0.8 h and an elimination half-life of about 26–38 h. Hepatic or renal failure does not influence serum concentrations.

Less than 10% of a given dose remains in the blood and most of this is bound to serum proteins (> 90%). Most of the remainder is thought to bind to cholesterol in host cell membranes. The highest amphotericin concentrations can be found in the liver, spleen, kidneys and lungs. Higher concentrations are achieved in the liver and spleen following administration of liposomal amphotericin (AmBisome). However, renal tissue concentrations are lower. Concentrations of the drug in peritoneal, pleural and joint fluids are about half the simultaneous concentration in serum. Levels in CSF are less than 5% of the simultaneous blood concentration.

3.2.5 Metabolism

No metabolites have been identified, but it is thought that amphotericin is metabolized in the liver. After treatment is discontinued the drug can be detected in the urine for at least 7 weeks. About 2–5% of a given dose is excreted unchanged in the urine.

3.2.6 Pharmaceutics

Amphotericin is available in oral, topical and parenteral forms.

Amphotericin is supplied for parenteral administration in lyophilized form in 50 mg amounts together with 41 mg of sodium deoxycholate (which acts as a dispersing agent) and a sodium phosphate buffer. The addition of 10 ml of sterile water gives a clear colloidal dispersion. This is further diluted with 490 ml of 5% dextrose solution prior to injection to give a final drug concentration of 100 mg/l. The dextrose solution should have a pH of 4.2 or greater to prevent precipitation of the drug. The diluted drug should be used within 24 h, but does not need to be protected from light. Other preparations for injection should not be added to an amphotericin infusion. If there are signs of precipitation, the infusion must be discarded.

Amphotericin is also supplied for parenteral administration encapsulated in liposomes (AmBisome). The drug is provided in lyophilized form in 50 mg amounts and is first reconstituted in 12 ml of cold (2–8°C) sterile water to give a drug concentration of 4 mg/ml. This solution is heated to 65°C for 10 min and allowed to cool to room temperature. The drug solution is further diluted with 5% dextrose solution to give a final drug concentration of 0.5 mg/ml and filter sterilized. The reconstituted drug in water can be stored in a refrigerator for up to 24 h prior to dilution with 5% dextrose solution. Infusion of the drug should be commenced within 6 h of dilution with 5% dextrose solution.

Other lipid-complexed formulations of amphotericin for parenteral administration are being developed.

**3.2.7
Therapeutic
use**

Topical amphotericin can be used to treat mucosal and cutaneous forms of candidosis.

Parenteral amphotericin is still the drug of choice for many forms of deep fungal infection, including aspergillosis, blastomycosis, candidosis, coccidioidomycosis, cryptococcosis, histoplasmosis, mucormycosis and paracoccidioidomycosis. Administration of the conventional formulation of the drug is inconvenient, necessitating prolonged intravenous access, and is associated with harmful side effects and unpleasant reactions which often limit the amount that can be given.

Liposomal amphotericin (AmBisome) is much better tolerated and much higher doses can be given with fewer toxic reactions. This formulation is indicated in patients who have failed to respond to conventional amphotericin, or in whom conventional amphotericin is considered to be contraindicated because of renal impairment.

The conventional parenteral formulation of amphotericin has been instilled into a number of sites, including the bladder, peritoneum and joints.

**3.2.8
Mode of
administration**

The dose and duration of topical treatment will differ from patient to patient and depend on the nature and extent of infection. The usual adult dose of the oral suspension for oral forms of candidosis is 1–2 ml (100–200 mg) at 6-h intervals. As the drug is not absorbed the success of treatment depends on maintaining an adequate concentration in the mouth for as long as possible. The recommended dosage of the oral suspension for infants and children is 1 ml (100 mg) at 6-h intervals.

Most patients with deep fungal infection are treated with 1–2 g of amphotericin over 6–10 weeks, but this will differ from person to person, depending upon the nature and extent of the infection and the underlying illness. In adults with normal renal function the usual dose of the conventional formulation of amphotericin is between 0.3 and 1.0 mg/kg. For empirical treatment the dose should be 1.0 mg/kg. There is no evidence to support the clinical prejudice that a lower dose can be used in suspected candidosis.

An initial test dose of 1 mg of amphotericin in 50 ml of dextrose solution should be given over 1–2 h (0.5 mg in children weighing less than 30 kg), with general clinical observation and monitoring of temperature, pulse and blood pressure at 30-min intervals. This is because occasional patients have an idiosyncratic reaction of severe hypotension or an anaphylaxis-like reaction. In the few patients with a reaction, the test infusion should be discontinued, suppor-

Table 3.1 Regimens for rapid escalation of amphotericin dosage

Time infusion started	Duration of infusion	Amphotericin dosage	Volume of solution 1	Volume of solution 2
0 h	2 h	1 mg	10 ml	40 ml
4 h	6 h	24 mg	240 ml	760 ml
16 h	6 h	25 mg	250 ml	750 ml
40 h	6 h	50 mg	500 ml	500 ml

(then at 24-h intervals, dose not to exceed 50 mg or 1.0 mg/kg per infusion, whichever is the lesser)

0 h	2 h	1 mg	10 ml	40 ml
2 h	6 h	9 mg	90 ml	360 ml
12 h	6 h	10 mg	100 ml	400 ml
24 h	6 h	20 mg	200 ml	300 ml
48 h	6 h	30 mg	300 ml	700 ml
72 h	6 h	40 mg	400 ml	600 ml
96 h	6 h	50 mg	500 ml	500 ml

(then at 24-h intervals; dose not to exceed 50 mg or 1.0 mg/kg per infusion whichever is the lesser)

Solution 1: amphotericin at 100 mg/l in 5% dextrose solution.
Solution 2: 5% dextrose solution.

tive treatment including hydrocortisone should be given, and a repeat test dose administered over a longer period. If the test dose is well tolerated, there can be progression to larger doses. Several dosage regimens are available (see Tables 3.1 and 3.2).

In patients who are not immunosuppressed or suffering a serious life-threatening infection, optimum dosage is best achieved through gradual augmentation of the dose. The dose can be increased up to 1.0 mg/kg, but individual infusions should not contain more than 50 mg of the drug.

In immunosuppressed patients and others with a serious infection, the dose of amphotericin should be increased as rapidly as the patient's tolerance of the drug will allow. Rapid augmentation of the dose carries a greater risk of acute renal failure, but immunosuppressed patients often tolerate these regimens well.

Four-hour infusions appear to be as well tolerated as the more traditional 6-h infusion period in patients with normal renal function. However, it is not advisable to give the infusion over less than 4 h.

After 2 weeks' treatment, blood concentrations become stable, tissue levels begin to accumulate and it becomes possible to administer the drug at 48- or 72-h intervals. The maximum dose can then be increased from 1.0 to 1.5 mg/kg.

The dosage of liposomal amphotericin (AmBisome) will also differ from patient to patient. It is usual to begin treatment with a dose of 1.0 mg/kg, but this can be increased to

Table 3.2 Regimen for gradual escalation of amphotericin dosage

Time infusion started	Duration of infusion	Amphotericin dosage	Volume of solution 1	Volume of solution 2
0 h	2 h	1 mg	10 ml	40 ml
2 h	6 h	9 mg	90 ml	360 ml
24 h	6 h	10 mg	100 ml	400 ml
48 h	6 h	20 mg	200 ml	300 ml
72 h	6 h	30 mg	300 ml	700 ml
96 h	6 h	40 mg	400 ml	600 ml
120 h	6 h	50 mg	500 ml	500 ml

(then at 24-h intervals; dose not to exceed 50 mg or 1.0 mg/kg per infusion whichever is the lesser)

Solution 1: amphotericin at 100 mg/l in 5% dextrose solution.
Solution 2: 5% dextrose solution.

3.0 mg/kg or even higher. This formulation is infused over a 30–60-min period.

In patients with meningitis due to *Coccidioides immitis*, intrathecal administration of amphotericin may be indicated (see Chapter 15). Intracisternal injection is to be preferred to lumbar intrathecal administration, because of the risk of chronic lumbar arachnoiditis. Injections should be given two or three times per week, with the dose increased from 0.025 mg as tolerated to 0.25–1.0 mg. Hydrocortisone sodium succinate (25 mg) should be added to the injection to reduce drug-induced inflammation.

Lower urinary tract candidosis will often respond to local treatment with amphotericin (see Chapter 11). Both continuous irrigation (50 mg/l in sterile water) and intermittent instillation (200–300 ml of a 50 mg/l solution at 6–8 h intervals) for 5–7 days have been used.

3.2.9
Adverse reactions

The immediate side effects of the intravenous infusion of amphotericin include fever, chills and rigors. These unpleasant reactions differ from patient to patient, but are most common during the first week of treatment and often diminish thereafter. These reactions can be prevented or lessened either by slowing the rate of infusion or by giving 25 mg of parenteral hydrocortisone just before the infusion is started or 25–50 mg during it if a reaction occurs. Parenteral chlorpheniramine (12.5–25 mg) or oral ibuprofen (10 mg/kg) can also reduce chills if given prior to the infusion.

Nausea and vomiting occur less often and, just as with fever and rigors, often diminish as treatment proceeds. Premedication with antiemetics is helpful.

Local phlebitis from intravenous administration of the conventional formulation of amphotericin is common. If the drug is given through a peripheral vein, the infusion site should be changed for each dose. Phlebitis can be prevented or ameliorated by slowing the rate of the infusion or by adding a small amount of heparin (500–1000 units/l) to the solution.

No serious immediate toxic reactions have so far been reported among individuals treated with liposomal amphotericin (AmBisome).

The most serious toxic effect of amphotericin is renal tubular damage. Most patients receiving the conventional formulation of the drug suffer some impairment of renal function, but it occurs most often in individuals given more than 0.5 mg/kg per day. Infants and children are less susceptible to the nephrotoxic effects of amphotericin. Renal function will return to almost normal levels in most patients several months after treatment has ceased, but irreversible renal failure can occur.

Renal damage can be reduced or prevented by careful monitoring during treatment. In the stable patient, renal function should be measured twice weekly and the treatment interrupted or the dosage modified if the serum creatinine concentration exceeds 250 μmol/l. Intravenous sodium supplementation may help to prevent amphotericin-induced renal impairment.

Patients who developed renal impairment while receiving the conventional formulation of amphotericin have improved or stabilized when liposomal amphotericin was substituted, even when the dose was increased.

Amphotericin also causes renal wasting of potassium and magnesium due to renal tubular damage and this can reach symptomatic proportions. Concentrations of these electrolytes should be monitored. Their loss can be reduced by administering 10–20 mg of oral amiloride per day, but intravenous electrolyte supplements must be given if low levels are seen.

Patients treated for more than 2 weeks often develop a mild normochromic, normocytic anaemia. Blood transfusion may be of benefit, but is not usually required.

Pulmonary reactions, with acute dyspnoea, hypoxaemia and interstitial infiltrates, can occur when treatment with amphotericin is combined with granulocyte transfusion. For this reason it is advisable to separate the infusion of the drug from the time of granulocyte transfusion.

3.2.10 Drug interactions

Amphotericin can augment the effects of other nephrotoxic drugs, such as aminoglycosides. Antineoplastic drugs can increase the nephrotoxic effects of amphotericin and these drugs should be administered together with great caution. Corticosteroids can increase amphotericin-induced potassium loss and the resulting hypokalaemia will enhance the action of digitalis glycosides.

3.3

Fluconazole

Fluconazole is a synthetic bis-triazole compound.

3.3.1
Mechanism of
action

Fluconazole inhibits the cytochrome P450-dependent 14α-demethylation step in the formation of ergosterol, the principal sterol in the membrane of susceptible fungal cells. The consequent depletion of ergosterol and accumulation of methylated sterols leads to alterations in a number of membrane-associated cell functions.

3.3.2
Spectrum of
action

Fluconazole has a broad spectrum of action including *Blastomyces dermatitidis, Coccidioides immitis, Cryptococcus neoformans, Histoplasma capsulatum* and *Paracoccidioides brasiliensis*. It is active against *Candida albicans, C. tropicalis* and *C. parapsilosis*, but many strains of *C. krusei* and *Torulopsis glabrata* (now reclassified as *C. glabrata*) appear to be insensitive. Fluconazole appears to be ineffective in aspergillosis and mucormycosis. It is active in dermatophytosis.

3.3.3
Acquired
resistance

This is rare, but resistant strains of *Candida albicans* have been recovered from AIDS patients receiving long-term treatment with fluconazole for oropharyngeal or oesophageal candidosis.

3.3.4
Pharmaco-
kinetics

In normal individuals, oral administration of fluconazole leads to rapid and almost complete absorption of the drug. Serum concentrations increase in proportion to dosage. Two hours after a single 50 mg oral dose, serum concentrations in the region of 1.0 mg/l can be anticipated, but after repeated dosing this increases to about 2.0–3.0 mg/l. Administration of the drug with food does not affect absorption.

Oral or parenteral administration of fluconazole results in rapid and widespread distribution of the drug. Unlike other azole antifungals, the protein binding of fluconazole is low (about 12%), resulting in high levels of circulating unbound drug. Levels of the drug in the CSF are between 50% and 90% of the simultaneous serum concentration. Levels in sputum and peritoneal fluid are similar to serum concentrations.

The main means of elimination is renal excretion of the unchanged drug. About 80% of an oral dose appears in the urine and concentrations of more than 100 mg/l have been attained in patients with normal renal function. The drug is cleared through glomerular filtration, but significant tubular reabsorption occurs. Fluconazole has a serum half-life of 25–30 h, but this is prolonged in renal failure, necessitating adjustment of the dosage regimen.

**3.3.5
Metabolism**

Unlike other azole antifungals, fluconazole is not metabolized in humans, but is excreted unchanged in the urine.

**3.3.6
Pharmaceutics**

Fluconazole is available in oral and parenteral forms.

The drug is supplied for parenteral administration in 100 ml amounts containing 2.0 mg/ml in 0.9% sodium chloride solution.

**3.3.7
Therapeutic use**

Fluconazole can be used to treat mucosal and cutaneous forms of candidosis. It is a useful drug in cryptococcal meningitis and can be used as maintenance treatment to prevent relapse of cryptococcosis in patients with AIDS. It is a promising drug for oral treatment of deep forms of candidosis, but should not be used as first-line treatment in neutropenic patients unless there are particular reasons for favouring it against established management.

**3.3.8
Mode of
administration**

As absorption following oral administration is good, this is the preferred method of administration. If the patient cannot take the drug by mouth, the intravenous solution can be used. This should be infused at a rate of 5–10 ml/min.

Vaginal candidosis can be treated with a single 150 mg oral dose of fluconazole. Oropharyngeal candidosis should be treated with 50–100 mg/d for 1–2 weeks. Oesophageal and mucocutaneous forms of candidosis and lower urinary tract candidosis require 50–100 mg/d for 2–4 weeks.

The recommended dose for patients with cryptococcosis or deep forms of candidosis is 400 mg on the first day followed by 200–400 mg/d. The duration of treatment will differ from patient to patient, depending upon the nature and extent of the infection and the underlying illness. At least 6–8 weeks is usually required for successful treatment of cryptococcosis. The recommended dose for children is 1–2 mg/kg for superficial forms of candidosis and 3–6 mg/kg for cryptococcosis or deep forms of candidosis.

Patients with renal impairment should be given the normal dose for the first 48 h of treatment. Thereafter, in persons with a creatinine clearance of 21–40 ml/min, the dosage interval should be doubled to 48 h or the dose halved. Persons with a clearance of 10–20 ml/min require a 72-h interval between doses.

Patients receiving regular dialysis require the usual dose after each dialysis session.

3.3.9
Adverse
reactions

Fluconazole is well tolerated. Minor side effects, such as nausea and vomiting, occur in a few patients. Transient elevations of liver function tests are quite common in AIDS patients treated with the drug. Unlike ketoconazole it does not affect adrenal or testicular steroid metabolism.

3.3.10
Drug
interactions

Fluconazole can augment the anticoagulant effect of warfarin. The serum half-life values of chlorpropamide, glibenclamide, glipizide and tolbutamide are prolonged. Phenytoin levels are elevated following concomitant administration with fluconazole. If both drugs are given together, phenytoin levels should be monitored and the dosage adjusted.

3.4

Flucytosine

Flucytosine (5-fluorocytosine) is a synthetic fluorinated pyrimidine.

3.4.1
Mechanism of
action

Flucytosine is transported into susceptible fungal cells by the action of cytosine permease and there converted by cytosine deaminase to 5-fluorouracil which is incorporated into RNA in place of uracil, with resulting abnormalities of protein synthesis. In addition, it blocks thymidylate synthetase causing inhibition of DNA synthesis.

3.4.2
Spectrum of
action

Flucytosine has a limited spectrum of action including *Candida* species, *Cryptococcus neoformans*, *Cladosporium carrionii*, *Fonsecaea* species and *Phialophora verrucosa*.

3.4.3
Acquired
resistance

A significant proportion of *Candida albicans* and *Cryptococcus neoformans* strains are resistant, both from the outset and emerging during treatment. The most common cause of resistance appears to be loss of the enzyme uridine monophosphate pyrophosphorylase.

3.4.4
Pharmaco-
kinetics

Flucytosine is well absorbed after oral administration, peak serum concentrations being reached about 2 h later. Absorption is slower in persons with impaired renal function but peak serum concentrations are higher. In adults with normal renal function a dose of 25 mg/kg given at 6-h intervals will produce peak serum concentrations of 70–80 mg/l and trough concentrations of 30–40 mg/l. The serum half-life is between 3 and 6 h, but is much longer in renal failure. There is slight accumulation of the drug during the first 4 days of treatment, but thereafter peak serum concentrations remain almost constant. Peak concentrations are reached in a shorter period of 1-2 h in persons who have received several previous doses of the drug. Following an intravenous infusion, blood concentrations similar to those attained after oral administration are obtained. Almost no protein binding occurs in serum.

Flucytosine is widely distributed, with CSF concentrations in the region of 75% of the simultaneous blood concentration. The main means of elimination is renal excretion of the unchanged drug. About 90% of an oral dose appears in the urine and concentrations of 1000 mg/l are not unusual in persons with normal renal function. The drug is retained in renal failure, necessitating modification of the dosage regimen.

3.4.5 Metabolism

Less than 1% of a dose of flucytosine is metabolized in humans. The drug is deaminated to 5-fluorouracil or dihydrofluorouracil and this could account for the myelotoxic effects associated with high serum concentrations. The remainder of the compound is excreted unchanged in the urine.

3.4.6 Pharmaceutics

Flucytosine is available as oral tablets and as an infusion for parenteral administration. The latter is supplied in 250 ml amounts containing 10 mg/ml in aqueous saline solution.

3.4.7 Therapeutic use

Flucytosine is seldom used as a single drug, other than in patients with certain forms of chromoblastomycosis. Its principal use is in combination with amphotericin in the treatment of cryptococcosis and deep forms of candidosis.

3.4.8 Mode of administration

As absorption following oral administration is good this is the preferred method of administration. If the patient cannot take the drug by mouth, the intravenous solution should be used. This can be administered through a venous catheter or as an intraperitoneal infusion. The drug should be infused over a 20–40-min period provided this is balanced with the fluid requirements of the patient. Twice-weekly blood counts (total white cells and platelets) should be performed.

In adults with normal renal function the usual starting dose of flucytosine is 50–150 mg/kg given as four divided doses at 6-h intervals. If renal function is impaired, an initial dose of 25 mg/kg should be given, but the subsequent dose and interval should be adjusted so as to produce peak serum concentrations of 70–80 mg/l and trough concentrations of 30–40 mg/l. The drug accumulates in renal failure necessitating modification of the dose regimen (see Table 3.3).

Table 3.3 Regimens for administration of flucytosine in renal impairment

Creatinine clearance (ml/min)	Individual dosage (mg/kg)	Dosage interval (h)
> 40	25–37.5	6
40–20	25–37.5	12
20–10	25–37.5	24
< 10	25–37.5	< 24*

Renal function is considered to be normal when creatinine clearance is greater than 40–50 ml/min or concentration of creatinine in serum is less than 180 µmol/l; concentration of creatinine in serum is not reliable unless renal function is stable.
* Dosage interval must be based on serum drug concentration measurement at frequent intervals.

**3.4.9
Adverse
reactions**

Abnormal elevations of liver function tests develop in about 5% of patients on flucytosine. Liver necrosis leading to or contributing to death occurred in two patients. Thrombocytopenia and leucopenia can occur if excessive serum concentrations are maintained. The effect is reversible if treatment is discontinued.

Many AIDS patients who receive flucytosine develop significant bone marrow suppression and the drug is best avoided.

The commonest symptomatic side effects are diarrhoea, nausea and vomiting.

**3.4.10
Drug
interactions**

The nephrotoxic effects of amphotericin result in elevated serum concentrations of flucytosine when these drugs are administered together.

3.5

Griseofulvin

Griseofulvin is an antifungal antibiotic derived from a number of *Penicillium* species. It was the first oral drug for treatment of dermatophytosis.

**3.5.1
Mechanism of
action**

Griseofulvin is a fungistatic drug which binds to microtubular proteins and inhibits fungal cell mitosis. It also acts as an inhibitor of nucleic acid synthesis.

**3.5.2
Spectrum of
action**

Griseofulvin has a limited spectrum of action which is almost restricted to the dermatophytes (*Epidermophyton floccosum, Microsporum* species and *Trichophyton* species). Its clinical use is limited to these infections. It is ineffective in cutaneous candidosis and pityriasis versicolor.

3.5.3 Acquired resistance

Treatment failure attributable to the development of griseofulvin resistance is an uncommon problem in patients with dermatophytoses.

3.5.4 Pharmaco-kinetics

Absorption of griseofulvin from the gastrointestinal tract is dependent on drug formulation. Administration of the drug with a high-fat meal will increase the rate and extent of absorption, but individual patients tend to achieve consistently high or low serum concentrations. Four hours after a single 500 mg dose, serum levels in the region of 0.5–2.0 mg/l can be anticipated.

Griseofulvin appears in the stratum corneum within 4–8 h of oral administration, as a result of drug secretion in perspiration. However, levels begin to fall soon after the drug is discontinued, and within 48–72 h it can no longer be detected.

3.5.5 Metabolism

Griseofulvin is metabolized by the liver to 6-desmethyl griseofulvin which is excreted in the urine. The drug has an elimination half-life from 9 to 21 h.

3.5.6 Pharmaceutics

Griseofulvin is available as oral tablets and oral suspension.

3.5.7 Therapeutic use

Griseofulvin is indicated in moderate to severe dermatophytoses of the skin, scalp hair, or nails where topical treatment is considered inappropriate or has failed.

3.5.8 Mode of administration

It is important to adjust the dose to the weight of the patient. The adult dose can range from 500 to 1000 mg either as a single or divided doses; not less than 10 mg/kg should be given. The dose for children under 25 kg is 10 mg/kg and 250–500 mg for children over 25 kg. It should be taken after meals.

The duration of treatment will differ from patient to patient and depend upon the nature and extent of the infection. For hair or skin at least 4 weeks' treatment is required. Long courses (usually 6–12 months) and high doses may be needed for nail infections. Long-term relapse rates are high; between 40% and 70% for toenails, but somewhat lower for fingernails.

3.5.9
Adverse
reactions

In most cases, prolonged courses and high doses are well tolerated. Patients have complained of headaches, nausea, vomiting and abdominal pain. Urticarial reactions and erythematous rashes occur in occasional patients.

The drug should be avoided in patients with liver disease.

3.5.10
Drug
interactions

Griseofulvin can diminish the anticoagulant effect of warfarin. Its absorption is reduced in patients receiving concomitant treatment with phenobarbitone.

3.6

Itraconazole

Itraconazole is a synthetic dioxolane triazole compound.

3.6.1
Mechanism of
action

Itraconazole interferes with the cytochrome P450-dependent 14α-demethylation step in the formation of ergosterol, the principal sterol in the fungal cell membrane. This leads to alterations in a number of membrane-associated cell functions.

3.6.2
Spectrum of
action

Itraconazole has a broad spectrum of action including *Aspergillus* species, *Blastomyces dermatitidis*, *Candida* species, *Coccidioides immitis*, *Cryptococcus neoformans*, *Histoplasma capsulatum* and *Paracoccidioides brasiliensis*. It is active in dermatophytosis and pityriasis versicolor.

3.6.3
Acquired
resistance

This has not been reported, but fluconazole- and ketoconazole-resistant *Candida albicans* strains have been cross-resistant to itraconazole.

3.6.4
Pharmaco-
kinetics

Absorption of itraconazole from the gastrointestinal tract is incomplete (about 55%), but is improved if the drug is given with food. Oral administration of a single 100 mg dose will produce peak serum concentration of between 0.1 and 0.2 mg/l about 2–4 h later. Much higher concentrations are obtained after repeated dosing, but there is much variation among individuals. Serum concentrations are reduced when gastric acid production is impaired.

Itraconazole is more than 99% protein-bound in serum. As a result, concentrations of the drug in fluids such as CSF are minimal. In contrast, drug concentrations in tissues, such as lung, liver and bone, are much higher than in serum.

Less than 0.03% of a given dose of itraconazole is excreted unchanged in the urine, but up to 18% is eliminated in faeces as unchanged drug.

3.6.5
Metabolism

Itraconazole is degraded in the liver into a large number of metabolites, most of which are inactive, and these are excreted with bile and urine. However, the major metabolite, hydroxyitraconazole, is bioactive. The serum half-life is about 20–30 h, increasing to 40 h after prolonged dosing.

3.6.6
Pharmaceutics

Itraconazole is available in an oral capsule form.

3.6.7
Therapeutic use

Itraconazole can be used to treat various superficial fungal infections, including the dermatophytoses, pityriasis versicolor, and oral and vaginal forms of candidosis. It appears to be a useful drug in blastomycosis, chromoblastomycosis, histoplasmosis, paracoccidioidomycosis and sporotrichosis and perhaps coccidioidomycosis as well. It is a promising drug for oral treatment of aspergillosis, cryptococcosis and deep forms of candidosis, but should not be used as first-line treatment in neutropenic patients unless there are particular reasons for favouring it against established management.

3.6.8
Mode of
administration

Vaginal candidosis can be treated with two 200 mg oral doses of itraconazole. Oropharyngeal candidosis can be treated with 100–200 mg/d for 2 weeks. Pityriasis versicolor requires 200 mg/d for 1 week. The recommended dose for patients with dermatophytoses is 100 mg/d for 2–4 weeks depending on the site of infection.

Initial reports suggest that dosages from 200 to 400 mg/d are effective in patients with subcutaneous or deep fungal infection. In neutropenic patients the dose should be increased to 400 mg/d to ensure adequate serum concentrations. It is recommended that a loading dose of 600 mg/d should be given for the first 4 days. Dosages above 200 mg/d should be given as two divided doses.

3.6.9
Adverse
reactions

Itraconazole is well tolerated. Minor side effects, such as nausea, headache and abdominal pain, occur in a few patients. Unlike ketoconazole it does not affect adrenal or testicular steroid metabolism.

Transient asymptomatic elevations of liver function tests have been seen in a few patients. It is advisable not to give the drug to patients with liver disease, or to patients who have experienced hepatotoxic reactions with other drugs.

3.6.10
Drug
interactions

Itraconazole concentrations are reduced following concomitant administration with phenytoin, rifampicin, antacids and H_2-antagonists. Terfenadine concentrations are elevated following concomitant administration with itraconazole and this has resulted in rare instances of life-threatening cardiac dysrhythmias. Cyclosporin and digoxin concentrations are also increased if these drugs are given together with itraconazole. It has been reported that itraconazole enhances the anticoagulant effect of warfarin.

3.7

Ketoconazole

Ketoconazole is a synthetic dioxolane imidazole compound.

3.7.1
Mechanism of
action

Like other azoles, it interferes with the biosynthesis of ergosterol, leading to alterations in a number of membrane-associated cell functions.

3.7.2
Spectrum of
action

Ketoconazole has a broad spectrum of action including *Blastomyces dermatitidis*, *Candida* species, *Coccidioides immitis*, *Histoplasma capsulatum* and *Paracoccidioides brasiliensis*. It is active in dermatophytosis and pityriasis versicolor, but only moderately effective in cryptococcosis and ineffective in aspergillosis and mucormycosis.

3.7.3
Acquired
resistance

This is rare, but resistant *Candida albicans* strains have been recovered from patients treated for chronic mucocutaneous candidosis and AIDS patients with oropharyngeal or oesophageal candidosis.

3.7.4
Pharmaco-
kinetics

Ketoconazole is not absorbed after topical application, but is well absorbed after oral administration, peak serum concentrations being reached 2–4 h later. Food delays absorption but does not significantly reduce the peak concentration. Two hours after a 400 mg dose serum concentrations in the region of 5–6 mg/l can be anticipated, but there is much variation among individuals. Much higher concentrations can be obtained with doses of 600–1000 mg. Penetration into CSF is poor and unreliable, although effective concentrations have been recorded with high doses (1200 mg) in some cases of meningitis. Less than 1% of an oral dose is excreted unchanged in the urine.

3.7.5
Metabolism

The drug is metabolized in the liver and the metabolites are excreted in the bile. None of the metabolites is active. The half-life appears to be dose-dependent. There is an initial half-life of 1 – 4 h and an elimination half-life ranging from 6 to 10 h.

3.7.6
Pharmaceutics

Ketoconazole is available in a number of oral and topical forms.

3.7.7
Therapeutic use

Ketoconazole remains a useful oral drug in chronic mucocutaneous candidosis and certain forms of histoplasmosis, blastomycosis and paracoccidioidomycosis. It should not be used for the oral treatment of dermatophytosis or cutaneous or vaginal candidosis, because of its possible effects on the liver and on steroid metabolism. However, it is a useful topical drug for dermatophytosis, cutaneous candidosis, pityriasis versicolor and seborrhoeic dermatitis.

3.7.8
Mode of
administration

Topical ketoconazole cream should be applied morning and evening and treatment should be continued for 48 h after all symptoms and signs have cleared. For those with pityriasis versicolor, the usual duration of treatment is 2 – 3 weeks. For dermatophytosis, 3 – 6 weeks treatment is required. Seborrhoeic dermatitis can be treated with ketoconazole shampoo twice per week for 2 – 4 weeks.

The usual adult oral dose is 200 – 400 mg/d depending on the infection being treated. In children a dose of 3 mg/kg can be used. The duration of treatment will depend upon the nature of the infection.

Ketoconazole requires an acid pH for absorption. If patients are receiving antacids, anticholinergics, or H_2-antagonists, these should be given at least 2 h after ketoconazole administration. In achlorhydric patients the tablets can be dissolved in 4 ml of 0.2 N hydrochloric acid before administration.

3.7.9
Adverse
reactions

Nausea and vomiting are the most common side effects. These occur in up to 50% of patients receiving oral doses of more than 800 mg, but can be reduced by giving the drug with food or at bedtime.

Transient minor elevations of liver function tests develop in about 5 – 10% of patients on oral ketoconazole. Treatment must be discontinued if these persist, if the abnormalities increase, or if symptoms associated with hepatic dysfunction appear.

The serious hepatotoxic side effects of ketoconazole are idiosyncratic and rare, occurring in between 1 : 10 000 and 1 : 15 000 patients. Most cases have been reported in patients treated for onychomycosis or chronic recalcitrant dermatophytosis. In most cases, hepatic damage is reversible when the drug is discontinued. Liver function tests must be performed before starting treatment and at frequent intervals thereafter, in particular in patients on prolonged treatment or in those receiving other hepatotoxic drugs.

High doses of ketoconazole block human steroid synthesis. Clinical manifestations of interference with testosterone synthesis sometimes occur. These include gynaecomastia, impotence and loss of hair. High-dose ketoconazole should be avoided in patients with tuberculosis, histoplasmosis, paracoccidioidomycosis or AIDS: these infections are often associated with hypoadrenalism and ketoconazole can aggravate this condition.

3.7.10
Drug
interactions

Concomitant administration of drugs that reduce gastric acid secretion (antacids, anticholinergics, H_2-antagonists) leads to reduced absorption of ketoconazole. Rifampicin reduces the blood concentrations of ketoconazole.

Ketoconazole prolongs the half-life of cyclosporin, leading to increased blood concentrations of that drug. Ketoconazole can augment the anticoagulant effect of warfarin.

3.8

Miconazole

Miconazole is a synthetic phenethyl imidazole compound.

3.8.1
Mechanism
of action

Like other azoles, miconazole interferes with the biosynthesis of ergosterol, leading to alterations in a number of membrane-associated cell functions. At high concentrations, miconazole interacts with membrane lipids causing direct membrane damage which results in leakage of cell constituents.

3.8.2
Spectrum of
action

Miconazole has a broad spectrum of action including *Aspergillus* species, *Candida* species, *Coccidioides immitis*, *Cryptococcus neoformans*, *Histoplasma capsulatum*, *Paracoccidioides brasiliensis* and *Pseudallescheria boydii*. It is also active in dermatophytosis.

3.8.3
Acquired
resistance

This is rare but *Candida albicans* strains resistant to ketoconazole have been cross-resistant to miconazole.

3.8.4
Pharmaco-
kinetics

Miconazole is not well absorbed following oral administration. Parenteral administration of a single 1000 mg dose will produce peak serum concentrations up to 7.5 mg/l.

There is rapid decline, with an initial serum half-life of 20–30 min and an elimination half-life of about 20 h. The drug is highly protein-bound in serum.

Miconazole concentrations in CSF are poor, but there is good penetration into peritoneal and joint fluid, and aqueous and vitreous humour. Less than 1% of a parenteral dose is excreted unchanged in the urine, but 40% of an oral dose is eliminated in faeces as unchanged drug.

3.8.5
Metabolism

Miconazole is metabolized in the liver and the metabolites are excreted in the bile and urine. None of the metabolites is active.

3.8.6
Pharmaceutics

Miconazole base is available in oral and parenteral forms. Miconazole nitrate is supplied in several forms for topical application.

The drug is supplied for parenteral administration in 20 ml amounts of cremophor containing 10 mg/ml. It must be diluted with sodium chloride solution or 5% dextrose solution.

3.8.7
Therapeutic use

Topical miconazole can be used to treat the dermatophytoses, and cutaneous and mucosal candidosis. Parenteral miconazole has been used to treat coccidioidomycosis and paracoccidioidomycosis. However, failure and relapse have been frequent problems. Its role in cryptococcosis and deep forms of candidosis remains unclear and it cannot now be recommended for these infections. It is ineffective in aspergillosis and mucormycosis, but is more active than amphotericin in the uncommon infection, pseudallescheriosis.

3.8.8
Mode of
administration

Vaginal candidosis can be treated with a 5 g dose of miconazole each night for 2 weeks, or 10 g can be administered for 1 week. Oral and oesophageal candidosis can be treated with oral tablets or the oral gel preparation. The usual adult dose is 250 mg at 6-h intervals. Treatment should be continued for 48 h after signs have cleared. For those with cutaneous dematophytosis, topical miconazole should be applied morning and evening until 2 weeks after the lesions have cleared. Cream containing miconazole nitrate and a steroid is useful in reducing inflammation.

The optimum dosage regimens for specific deep fungal infections or sites of infection have not been established. The adult dose can range from 200 to 1200 mg per infusion diluted in 200–500 ml of fluid. The usual adult dose is 600 mg given at 8-h intervals. The infusion must be given over a period of not less than 30 min. In children the recommended dose is 20–40 mg/kg per day. A dose of 15 mg/kg per infusion must not be exceeded. The duration of treatment will depend upon the infection and the underlying illness of the patient.

3.8.9
Adverse
reactions

Topical miconazole can cause local irritation. Oral forms of the drug have caused mild gastrointestinal upsets. The commonest symptomatic side effects of parenteral miconazole have included nausea, vomiting, fever, rash, drowsiness, diarrhoea and anorexia.

Phlebitis has been reported in about 30% of patients receiving miconazole through a peripheral vein. Intense pruritus has occurred in 25% of patients and has necessitated discontinuation of the drug in some individuals.

Rapid injection of miconazole can produce transient tachycardia or cardiac arrhythmia. These effects, if not transient, respond to lignocaine.

3.8.10
Drug
interactions

Miconazole intravenous solution may augment the anticoagulant effect of warfarin. It may also potentiate the effect of hypoglycaemic drugs.

3.9

Terbinafine

Terbinafine is a synthetic allylamine compound.

3.9.1
Mechanism of
action

Terbinafine inhibits the action of squalene epoxidase, a crucial enzyme in the formation of ergosterol, the principal sterol in the membrane of susceptible fungal cells. The consequent accumulation of squalene leads to membrane disruption and cell death.

3.9.2
Spectrum of
action

Terbinafine is effective against the dermatophytes (*Epidermophyton floccosum*, *Microsporum* species and *Trichophyton* species) and its clinical use is presently limited to these infections. Although it has also been shown to be active against *Aspergillus* species, *Blastomyces dermatitidis*, *Cryptococcus neoformans* and *Histoplasma capsulatum* in vitro, it is not effective in vivo. It is fungistatic for *Candida albicans* but fungicidal for some other *Candida* species including *C. parapsilosis*.

3.9.3
Acquired
resistance

This has not been reported.

3.9.4 Pharmacokinetics

About 5% of a given dose of terbinafine is absorbed following topical application. The drug is well absorbed (> 70%) after oral administration. Two hours after a single 250 mg oral dose, serum concentrations in the region of 0.8–1.5 mg/l can be anticipated. Levels increase in proportion to dosage up to at least 750 mg.

Terbinafine is a lipophilic drug which appears to concentrate in the dermis, epidermis and adipose tissue. It appears in the stratum corneum within a few hours of oral administration being commenced, as a result of secretion in sebum. It has been detected in the distal portion of nails after 4 weeks' treatment, indicating that diffusion from the nail bed is a major factor in drug penetration.

3.9.5 Metabolism

Terbinafine is metabolized by the liver and the inactive metabolites are excreted in the urine. The drug has an elimination half-life of 17 h, but this is prolonged in patients with hepatic or renal impairment.

3.9.6 Pharmaceutics

Terbinafine (as hydrochloride) is available in oral and topical forms.

3.9.7 Therapeutic use

Oral terbinafine can be used to treat dermatophytoses of the skin and nails where topical treatment is considered inappropriate or has failed.

It is ineffective against pityriasis versicolor.

3.9.8 Mode of administration

The usual adult dose is one 250 mg oral tablet per day. The duration of treatment will depend upon the site and extent of infection (see Chapter 4). For foot infections 2–6 weeks' treatment is required.

The dose should be halved in patients with impaired hepatic or renal function (creatinine clearance less than 50 ml/min or serum creatinine concentration more than 300 µmol/ml).

3.9.9 Adverse reactions

Terbinafine is well tolerated. The commonest side effects are nausea and abdominal pain, and allergic skin reactions, but these are often mild and transient. Loss of taste has been reported. No life-threatening reactions have occurred.

3.9.10 Drug interactions

Terbinafine concentrations are reduced following concomitant administration with rifampicin, and increased if given together with cimetidine.

3.10	**Other compounds for topical administration** In addition to the antifungal compounds described so far, a number of other drugs are available for topical use.
3.10.1 Amorolfine	Morpholine compound used for the treatment of fungal nail infections.
3.10.2 Bifonazole	Imidazole compound used for the treatment of the dermatophytoses and pityriasis versicolor.
3.10.3 Clotrimazole	Imidazole compound used for the treatment of the dermatophytoses and oral, cutaneous and genital candidosis.
3.10.4 Econazole nitrate	Imidazole compound used for the treatment of the dermatophytoses and oral, cutaneous and genital candidosis. It has also been used to treat corneal infections.
3.10.5 Isoconazole nitrate	Imidazole compound used for the treatment of vaginal candidosis.
3.10.6 Naftifine	Allylamine compound used for the treatment of the dermatophytoses.
3.10.7 Natamycin	Polyene compound used for the treatment of oral and vaginal candidosis. It has also been used to treat corneal infections.
3.10.8 Nystatin	Polyene compound used for the treatment of oral, cutaneous and mucosal forms of candidosis. It has also been used to treat corneal infections.
3.10.9 Sulconazole nitrate	Imidazole compound used for the treatment of the dermatophytoses and cutaneous candidosis.
3.10.10 Tioconazole	Imidazole compound used for the treatment of the dermatophytoses (including nail infections) and cutaneous and vaginal candidosis.
3.11	**Empirical treatment of suspected fungal infection in the neutropenic patient** Treatment of established candidosis or aspergillosis in the neutropenic patient is often unsuccessful. For this reason it is often better to begin antifungal treatment without waiting

for formal proof that a neutropenic patient with persistent fever ($>$ 72–96 h duration), resistant to antibacterial drugs, has a fungal infection. In this situation amphotericin must be used.

Empirical treatment should be initiated with the usual test dose (1 mg) of amphotericin. If possible, the full therapeutic dosage level (1.0 mg/kg per day) should be reached within the first 24 h of treatment. There is no need for gradual escalation of dosage, nor is there evidence to support the clinical prejudice that a lower dose can be used in suspected candidosis.

The duration of treatment will differ from patient to patient. If the patient responds and a diagnosis of fungal infection is established, a full course of treatment (1.5–2.0 g over 6–12 weeks) should be given. More often, however, the patient responds and/or the neutrophil count recovers, but a firm diagnosis is not obtained. In this situation it is reasonable to discontinue amphotericin when the neutrophil count exceeds 0.5×10^9 per litre, the fever resolves, other relevant symptoms and signs resolve, and relevant radiological abnormalities return to normal. Although there is no direct evidence to support the clinical prejudice that supected aspergillosis requires a longer period of treatment than suspected candidosis, this common practice is justified.

Neutropenic patients who recover from a deep fungal infection, such as aspergillosis, often suffer from reactivation of the infection during subsequent periods of immunosuppression. One solution to this problem is to begin empirical treatment with amphotericin (1 mg/kg per day) not less than 48 h before antileukaemic treatment is commenced. This drug should be continued until the neutrophil count has recovered.

3.12

Prophylactic treatment for prevention of fungal infection

There have been numerous attempts to develop regimens that will reduce intestinal and oral colonization with *Candida* species and help prevent oral candidosis. There have, however, been no convincing demonstrations that either nystatin or amphotericin oral suspensions or tablets prevent the development of oral, oesophageal or deep forms of candidosis in neutropenic patients. Their use alone is not recommended.

Oral ketoconazole does appear to reduce the incidence of oral candidosis and oesophagitis in neutropenic patients;

whether it prevents deep candidosis is less clear. If offers no protection against aspergillosis or mucormycosis and its use can lead to the selection of less sensitive *Candida glabrata* strains in the gastrointestinal tract. It is not well absorbed in bone marrow transplant (BMT) recipients. Moreover, it prolongs the half-life of cyclosporin and leads to increased serum concentrations of that drug. Its use as prophylaxis in organ transplant or BMT recipients is therefore not recommended.

Fluconazole (50 mg/d) has been shown to reduce the incidence of oral and faecal colonization and oral infection with all *Candida* species apart from *C. glabrata* and *C. krusei*. However, it offers no protection against aspergillosis or mucormycosis. Fluconazole does not affect cyclosporin levels and it can be recommended as an effective drug for prevention of candidosis in neutropenic patients.

Itraconazole (400 mg/d) does appear to help prevent the development of aspergillosis, but not mucormycosis, in neutropenic patients. However, erratic absorption of the drug from the gastrointestinal tract is a problem. Its use is recommended in units where patients are nursed without high-efficiency particulate air (HEPA) filters, where there is a high incidence of aspergillosis, or where building works are being undertaken. Itraconazole should be substituted for fluconazole prophylaxis in such institutions in patients who have been neutropenic for longer than 3 weeks.

3.13 Laboratory monitoring

3.13.1 Amphotericin

The results of minimal inhibitory concentration (MIC) determinations with amphotericin are less subject to test conditions than is the case with most other antifungal drugs. Most strains of most of the principal human pathogens are inhibited from growth at concentrations ranging from 0.05 to 1.0 mg/l. These concentrations are similar to blood levels attained during parenteral treatment, but it is unsafe to assume that all patients will respond to the drug. Other factors, such as the immunological status of the patient and the location of the infection, must be taken into account. There is usually no need to test isolates of *Aspergillus* species, *Candida* species or *Cryptococcus neoformans* before starting treatment, because insensitive strains are rare. Isolates from patients with a serious infection that does not respond as expected to amphotericin should be tested.

Many isolates of *Trichosporon beigelii* (*T. cutaneum*) and

Pseudallescheria boydii are resistant to amphotericin with MICs in excess of 2.0 mg/l. There is no need to determine MICs with the aetiological agents of mucormycosis: the results have not been correlated with clinical outcome, but amphotericin is the only antifungal drug effective in these infections.

Monitoring of amphotericin serum concentrations during treatment is not indicated. The question of the optimum serum concentration of the drug for a particular fungal infection has not been resolved. Although amphotericin is nephrotoxic, high blood concentrations do not lead to greater impairment of renal function, nor does renal failure result in higher blood concentrations.

3.13.2
Fluconazole

The results of MIC tests with fluconazole are highly dependent on the conditions of the test, being markedly affected by the concentration of the fungal inoculum, the composition and pH of the medium, and the temperature and length of incubation. As a consequence it is not unusual to obtain MICs for responsive organisms that are much higher than concentrations of drug attainable in vivo. However, high MICs have sometimes been correlated with clinical failure or relapse.

There is no need to test the susceptibility of isolates of *Cryptococcus neoformans* or *Candida albicans* before starting treatment. However, if treatment failure or relapse occurs despite adequate serum concentrations of fluconazole, the MICs of the drug for recent isolates from the patient should be compared with those of earlier isolates and sensitive and resistant reference organisms.

In general, serum concentrations of fluconazole are more predictable than those of other azole drugs and there is no need for their measurement. Excessive concentrations have not so far been associated with unwanted side effects. Concentrations are unchanged in patients with AIDS and in BMT recipients, and the reduction in concentration following concomitant administration with rifampicin is smaller than that seen with other azole antifungals, such as ketoconazole.

3.13.3
Flucytosine

The major disadvantage of this drug is the fact that a significant proportion of *Candida albicans* and *Cryptococcus neoformans* isolates are resistant with MICs in excess of 16 mg/l. For this reason, isolates from all patients destined to receive the drug on its own should be tested, as should isolates recovered during treatment.

Serum concentrations of flucytosine should be measured in all patients; this is essential when there is renal impairment or when the drug is given in combination with amphotericin, to ensure adequate therapeutic concentrations and avoid excessive concentrations that can cause toxic effects.

Levels should be determined twice weekly or more frequently if renal function is changing. Blood should be taken just before a dose of flucytosine is due, and 2 h after an oral dose or 30 min after an intravenous dose. In patients with renal impairment peak concentrations tend to occur later after oral dosing.

3.13.4 Itraconazole

As with fluconazole, the results of MIC tests are highly dependent on the conditions under which the tests are performed, and it is not unusual to obtain MICs for responsive organisms that are higher than the concentrations of drug attainable in vivo. Should treatment failure or relapse occur despite adequate serum concentrations of the drug, the MICs of recent isolates from the patient should be compared with those of earlier isolates and sensitive and resistant reference organisms.

Absorption of itraconazole after oral administration shows marked variation between individuals. Low concentrations can be anticipated in AIDS and BMT patients, and in patients receiving concomitant treatment with rifampicin. Low serum concentrations of itraconazole (less than 0.25 mg/l at 4 h) may predict failure of treatment. Levels should be measured in patients with life-threatening fungal infections, in patients in whom poor absorption or drug interactions are anticipated, and when there is treatment failure or relapse. High serum concentrations have not so far been associated with unwanted side effects.

Serum concentrations should be determined only after the patient has reached the steady state, typically after 1–2 weeks. Blood should be taken 4 h after an oral dose. High-performance liquid chromatography (HPLC) is the preferred method for determining itraconazole concentrations because microbiological methods detect an active metabolite in addition to the drug itself.

3.13.5 Ketoconazole

As with the other azoles, the results of MIC tests are highly dependent on test conditions and it is not unusual to obtain MICs for responsive organisms that are higher than the concentrations of drug attainable in vivo. Should treatment failure or relapse occur despite adequate serum concentrations, the actions described for fluconazole and itraconazole should be taken.

Routine determination of serum concentrations is not required. Low concentrations can be anticipated in patients with AIDS and in BMT recipients. Drug concentrations are reduced by concomitant administration of antacids, H_2-receptor antagonists and rifampicin. Low concentrations have been associated with therapeutic failure and it is important to measure the concentration of the drug if this is suspected. The hepatotoxic side effects of ketoconazole are not associated with high serum concentrations.

4 Dermatophytosis

4.1

Introduction

The term dermatophytosis is used to describe infections of the skin, hair and nails due to a group of related filamentous fungi, the dermatophytes, which are also known as the ringworm fungi.

The clinical presentation of these infections depends on several factors including: the site of infection, the immunological response of the host and the species of infecting fungus. In most forms of dermatophytosis, the fungus is confined to the superficial stratum corneum, nails and hair. However, deeper infection involving the dermis can occur, as in kerion, and this can result in the formation of suppurative lesions.

4.2

The causal organisms and their habitat

There are three genera of dermatophytes, *Trichophyton*, *Microsporum* and *Epidermophyton*. Of the 40 or so species that are recognized at present, some are worldwide in distribution, but others are restricted to particular continents or regions. About 10 species are common causes of human infection.

The dermatophytes are termed geophilic, zoophilic or anthropophilic depending upon whether their normal habitat is the soil, an animal or man. Members of all three groups can cause human infection, but their different natural reservoirs have important epidemiological implications in relation to the acquisition, site and spread of human infection.

Although the geophilic group of dermatophytes can cause infection in both animals and humans, their normal habitat is the soil. Members of the anthropophilic and zoophilic groups are thought to have evolved from these and other keratinophilic soil-inhabiting fungi, different species having adapted to different natural hosts. Individual members of the zoophilic group are often associated with a particular animal host, for instance *M. canis* with cats and dogs and *T. verrucosum* with cattle. However, these organisms can also spread to humans.

Those dermatophytes for whom humans are the usual host are termed anthropophilic. These species can be divided into those which are common causes of scalp infections, for instance *M. audouinii* and *T. tonsurans*, and those which cause foot and nail infections, for instance *E. floccosum* and *T. rubrum*.

4.3

Laboratory diagnosis of dermatophytosis

It has been estimated that as much as 50% of suspicious material sampled from infected persons may not contain any fungus. It is important, therefore, to employ the correct procedures when taking specimens for laboratory investigation.

It is helpful to clean the lesion with 70% alcohol before taking the specimen; this improves the chances of detecting the fungus microscopically. Prior cleaning is essential if ointments, creams or powders have been applied to the lesion.

Material is best collected into, and transported in, folded squares of black paper. This permits drying of the specimen which helps to reduce bacterial contamination and also provides conditions under which specimens may easily be stored for long periods.

Microscopic examination and culture of clinical specimens should both be attempted on all occasions.

The recognition of fungal hyphae and/or arthrospores during microscopic examination of clinical material is sufficient for the diagnosis of dermatophytosis but, apart from hair specimens, gives no indication as to the species of fungus involved. With hair the size and arrangement of the arthrospores can indicate which group of species is involved.

Culture is a more reliable diagnostic procedure than microscopic examination. Because it permits the species of fungus involved to be determined, it can provide information as to the source of the infection and aid the selection of the most appropriate form of treatment.

It is not unusual to isolate moulds other than dermatophytes from abnormal skin and nails. In many cases, these are casual, transient contaminants and direct microscopic examination of clinical material is negative. However, certain moulds are capable of causing infection and, when this is so, it is important that their significance is recognized. These infections are described in Chapters 6 and 7.

4.4

Tinea capitis

4.4.1
Definition

The term tinea capitis is used to refer to dermatophyte infections of the scalp and hair.

**4.4.2
Geographical
distribution**

The condition is worldwide in distribution, but is most prevalent in Africa, Asia and southern and eastern Europe, where it is the commonest form of dermatophytosis. Improved standards of hygiene and prompt eradication of sporadic infection have led to a marked decline in the incidence of tinea capitis in North America and western Europe. Favus used to be worldwide in distribution, but is now confined to North Africa, the Middle East and parts of southern and eastern Europe.

**4.4.3
Causative
agents**

Tinea capitis is caused by a number of *Trichophyton* and *Microsporum* species. *M. canis* is a frequent cause of the condition in western Europe, but *T. violaceum* is predominant in eastern and southern Europe and North Africa. *T. tonsurans* is predominant in North America.

Tinea capitis due to anthropophilic *Microsporum* species is a contagious disease endemic in many countries. It is primarily a disease of children, being more common in males than females, and most prevalent between 6 and 10 years of age. The disease seldom persists beyond the age of 16. Large outbreaks often occur in schools or other places where children are congregated. The zoophilic *Microsporum* species and *Trichophyton* species are seldom responsible for more than minor outbreaks of human infection. Household pets, such as dogs and cats, are a common source of infection, but feral cats are another prolific source of *M. canis*.

Tinea capitis due to anthropophilic *Trichophyton* species is another contagious disease. It is most common in male children, under the age of 12.

T. schoenleinii is considered to be the sole aetiological agent of favus, although infections with other dermatophytes, such as *M. gypseum*, *T. verrucosum* and *T. violaceum*, can sometimes produce somewhat similar lesions. Although *T. schoenleinii* is an anthropophilic dermatophyte, favus is less contagious than other forms of tinea capitis due to *Microsporum* or other *Trichophyton* species. It is usually contracted in childhood and may persist into adult life. Debilitated or malnourished children, or children suffering from a chronic disease such as tuberculosis, are more susceptible to this infection. Instances have been reported in which several generations of the same family were affected.

**4.4.4
Clinical
manifestations**

The clinical manifestations of tinea capitis are varied and can range from mild scaling lesions (similar to seborrhoeic dermatitis), to widespread alopecia or, less commonly, to a highly inflammatory suppurating lesion termed a kerion. The latter condition is usually caused by infection with a zoophilic dermatophyte.

M. canis and *M. equinum* (both acquired from infected animals), and *M. audouinii* and *M. ferrugineum* (both acquired from infected humans) invade the scalp hair in a distinctive manner. The lesions consist of one or more discrete, round or oval, erythematous patches of scaling and hair loss (2–6 cm in diameter). These may extend with time to involve the entire scalp. The hairs in these lesions are all parasitized and most of them are broken about 2–3 mm above the surface of the scalp. The hair surface is covered with a dense mass of small (2–3 μm diameter) arthrospores. Infected hairs show green fluorescence under Wood's light.

T. mentagophytes and *T. verrucosum* infections of the scalp are acquired from infected animals. The typical lesions are single and are erythematous and pustular. Kerion formation is common. Infected hairs are covered with chains of large spores and are not fluorescent under Wood's light.

T. tonsurans, *T. violaceum* and *T. soudanense* infections are acquired from infected humans. The typical lesions are erythematous, irregular patches of scaling (0.5–1.0 cm in diameter). The lesions are not well demarcated. The affected hairs often break off at the scalp surface, leading to alopecia and giving a black-dot appearance in dark-haired patients. Other hairs are broken off 1–2 mm from the scalp surface and are often obscured under a layer of scales. Infected hairs are filled with arthrospores and do not fluoresce under Wood's light.

The main clinical manifestations of favus are the formation of crusted, inflamed patches on the scalp, with permanent hair loss due to follicular scarring. The scalp itches and gives off a foetid odour. The crusts (scutula) develop around the follicular openings and can fuse to cover large areas of the scalp. Long-standing favus can lead to permanent diffuse patches of alopecia. Although infected, the hairs tend not to break off, and can grow to normal length. Infected hairs give off a dull green fluorescence under Wood's light.

4.4.5
Differential diagnosis

Tinea capitis is often difficult to distinguish from other causes of scaling (such as psoriasis and seborrhoeic dermatitis) or hair loss (such as alopecia areata and discoid lupus erythematosus). For this reason, Wood's light examination and laboratory tests should be performed in any patient with scaling scalp lesions or hair loss of undetermined origin.

**4.4.6
Essential
investigations
and their
interpretation**

Specimens from the scalp should include hair roots, the contents of plugged follicles and skin scales. Except for favus, the distal portion of infected hair seldom contains any fungus. For this reason, cut hairs without roots are unsuitable for mycological investigation. One method which is useful for collecting material from the scalp is hairbrush sampling.

Direct microscopic examination of infected material should reveal arthrospores of the fungus located outside (ectothrix) or inside (endothrix) the affected hair. The arthrospores can be either small ($2-4\,\mu m$ in diameter) or large (up to $10\,\mu m$ in diameter) in size. Skin scales will contain hyphae and arthrospores.

In *T. schoenleinii* infection (favus), loose chains of arthrospores and air spaces are seen within the affected hairs. The scutulum (crust) consists of mycelium, neutrophils and epidermal cells.

Isolation of the aetiological agent in culture will permit the species of fungus involved to be determined. This will provide information as to the source of the infection and aid the selection of appropriate treatment.

Hairs infected with *M. audouinii* and *M. canis* produce a brilliant green fluorescence under Wood's light in a darkened room. However, in recent infections, or at the spreading margin of lesions, the fluorescent part of the hair may not yet have emerged from the follicle and fluorescence can only be detected after the hair is plucked. *T. schoenleinii* causes a pale dull green fluorescence of infected hair. The fluorescent hairs tend to be long, in contrast to the short hair stumps characteristic of microsporum infection.

It is important to remember that creams and ointments applied to scalp lesions, as well as host tissue and exudates, can produce a pale bluish or purplish fluorescence under Wood's light.

**4.4.7
Management**

If possible, specimens for mycological examination should be taken before starting treatment. If oral treatment is being considered, mycological confirmation of the clinical diagnosis is essential before treatment is commenced.

Various topical imidazole preparations can be used to treat tinea capitis, including clotrimazole, miconazole and sulconazole. These drugs are safe and side effects after local application are uncommon.

The drug of choice for tinea capitis is oral griseofulvin. The usual adult dose is 500 mg/d given after food, but this can be increased to 1000 mg/d. Not less than 10 mg/kg should be given. The dose for children over 25 kg is 250–500 mg/d. Those weighing less than 25 kg should be given 10 mg/kg. The duration of treatment depends on the nature of the infection and the clinical response, but 2–3 months is usually required. Mycological tests should be repeated 1 month after starting treatment and again before discontinuing the drug.

Itraconazole (100 mg/d for about 2 weeks) and terbinafine (250 mg/d for about 2 weeks) appear promising, but are not at present licensed for the oral treatment of tinea capitis.

To prevent epidemics of anthropophilic tinea capitis due to *M. audouinii* from developing, all contacts of infected children should be examined with Wood's light. Patients should be kept away from school until the infection has cleared.

4.5	**Tinea corporis**

**4.5.1
Definition**

The term tinea corporis is used to refer to dermatophyte infections of the trunk, legs and arms, but excluding the groin, hands and feet.

**4.5.2
Geographical
distribution**

The condition is worldwide in distribution, but is most prevalent in tropical and subtropical regions.

**4.5.3
Causative
agents**

Tinea corporis is caused by *Epidermophyton floccosum* and many species of *Trichophyton* and *Microsporum*. Infection with anthropophilic species, such as *E. floccosum* or *T. rubrum* often follows autoinoculation from another infected body site, such as the feet. Tinea corporis caused by *T. tonsurans* is occasionally, but increasingly, being seen in children with tinea capitis and their close contacts.

Tinea corporis commonly occurs following contact with infected household pets or farm animals, but occasional cases result from contact with wild mammals or contaminated soil. *M. canis* is a frequent cause of human infection, and *T. verrucosum* infection is common in rural areas. Human-to-human spread of infection with geophilic or zoophilic species is unusual.

**4.5.4
Clinical
manifestations**

Tinea corporis may affect any body site, but is more likely to occur on exposed parts. Patients may complain of mild pruritus. The clinical manifestations are variable, depending on the species of fungus involved and the extent of progression, but in typical cases, round scaling lesions which are dry, erythematous and clearly circumscribed, are seen. The fungus is more active at the margin of the lesions and hence this is more erythemato-squamous than the middle, which tends to heal earlier. As the first ring of advancing infection continues to spread outwards, it may become surrounded by one or more concentric rings or arcuate patterns. Adjacent lesions may fuse producing gyrate patterns. In some instances, particularly when a zoophilic dermatophyte is involved, the lesion may be markedly inflamed and even pustular.

The lesions are often more extensive in immunosuppressed individuals.

Patients with tinea corporis often have coexistent dermatophytosis of the scalp, beard or nails. In these cases, the smooth skin infection may be the primary site, or it may have been derived from lesions elsewhere.

4.5.5
Differential
diagnosis

Tinea corporis can be difficult to distinguish from other causes of erythematous, scaling skin lesions, such as contact dermatitis, eczema, pityriasis rosea and psoriasis. For this reason, laboratory tests should be performed in any patient with skin lesions of undetermined origin.

4.5.6
Essential
investigations
and their
interpretation

Material for mycological investigation should be collected from the raised border of the lesion by scraping outwards with a glass microscope slide or blunt scalpel held perpendicular to the skin. If vesicles are present, the entire top should be submitted for examination.

Direct microscopic examination of infected material should reveal the branching hyphae characteristic of a dermatophyte infection.

Isolation of the aetiological agent in culture will permit the species of fungus involved to be determined. This will provide information as to the source of the infection and aid the selection of appropriate treatment. Treatment of an infected animal is essential to prevent spread to further individuals.

4.5.7
Management

Topical antifungal preparations are the treatment of choice for localized lesions. Various imidazole and allylamine compounds are available in a number of topical formulations. All give similar high cure rates (70–100%) and side effects are uncommon. These drugs should be applied morning and evening for at least 2–4 weeks. Treatment should be continued for at least 1 week after the lesions have cleared and the medication should be applied at least 3 cm beyond the advancing margin of the lesion.

If the lesions are extensive or the patient fails to respond to topical preparations, oral treatment is usually indicated. The drug of first choice is griseofulvin (500–1000 mg/d) and this may usefully be given in combination with topical treatment. Oral treatment with itraconazole (100 mg/d for 2 weeks) or terbinafine (250 mg/d for 4 weeks) has also proved effective.

4.6 Tinea cruris

4.6.1 Definition

The term tinea cruris is used to refer to dermatophyte infections of the groin and pubic region.

4.6.2 Geographical distribution

The condition is worldwide in distribution.

4.6.3 Causative agents

The dermatophytes most often encountered in tinea cruris are *E. floccosum* and *T. rubrum*.

Tinea cruris is a common form of dermatophytosis. It is more prevalent in men than women. It usually occurs between the ages of 18 and 60, but is most prevalent between the ages of 18 and 25, and between 40 and 50.

Maceration and occlusion of the skin in the groin give rise to warm moist conditions that favour the development of the infection.

Tinea cruris is commonly acquired from another infected area of the same individual. Autoinoculation from infected feet via towels is not uncommon.

Tinea of the groin is a highly contagious condition and minor epidemics often occur in schools and other communities. The infection is usually transmitted via contaminated towels or the floors of bathrooms, showers, or hotel bedrooms, etc.

4.6.4 Clinical manifestations

Tinea cruris usually presents as one or more rapidly spreading, erythematous lesions with central clearing on the inside of the thighs. The lesions, which tend to coalesce, have a raised erythematous border which encloses a blackish-brown area of scaling. Patients often complain of intense pruritus. Scratching may result in small satellite lesions which sometimes fuse with the primary lesion altering its outline.

The infection may spread from the inside of the thigh to the scrotum, penis, natal cleft and gluteal folds, as well as to the anterior and posterior aspects of the thighs. Localized scrotal infection is quite common: the clinical signs are often inconspicuous.

Tinea of the groin may also spread to other skin folds, particularly to the axillae, which may also be the primary site of infection. Interdigital infection of the hands or feet may also develop secondarily from the groin infection. Infection of the toe clefts may precede the development of tinea cruris.

4.6.5
Differential diagnosis

Tinea cruris can be difficult to distinguish from other causes of erythematous groin lesions, such as bacterial and candidal intertrigo, erythrasma, psoriasis and sebhorrhoeic dermatitis. For this reason, laboratory tests should be performed in any patient with groin lesions of undetermined origin.

4.6.6
Essential investigations and their interpretation

Direct microscopic examination of infected material should reveal the branching hyphae characteristic of a dermatophyte infection. Isolation of the aetiological agent in culture will permit the species of fungus involved to be determined.

4.6.7
Management

Most patients with tinea cruris will respond to local anti-fungal treatment within 2–4 weeks. Topical imidazole compounds, such as clotrimazole, econazole, miconazole and sulconazole, should be applied morning and evening for at least 2 weeks. To prevent relapse treatment should be continued for at least 2 weeks after the disappearance of all symptoms and signs of infection.

If a patient has extensive infection (involving the buttocks or anterior or posterior aspects of the thighs, for instance) or tinea pedis as well, oral griseofulvin (500–1000 mg/d for 2–6 weeks) should be given in addition to topical treatment. Folliculitis is another indication for the addition of an oral agent.

Oral treatment with itraconazole (100 mg/d for 2 weeks) or terbinafine (250 mg/d for 2–4 weeks) should be considered for use in patients with chronic, recalcitrant tinea cruris that is unresponsive to griseofulvin.

To prevent reinfection following treatment, the patient

should be advised to dry the groin thoroughly after bathing and to use separate towels to dry the groin and the rest of the body. The feet should be examined and treated if tinea pedis is present. Occlusive or synthetic garments should be avoided. If the patient is obese, weight loss may be of benefit by reducing chafing and sweating.

Tinea cruris recurs in about 20–25% of patients. If this happens, patients should be given further topical antifungal treatment and advice about nonpharmacological control measures should be repeated.

4.7	**Tinea pedis**

4.7.1 Definition	The term tinea pedis is used to refer to dermatophyte infections of the feet. These infections often involve the interdigital spaces, but chronic diffuse desquamation can affect the entire sole.

4.7.2 Geographical distribution	The condition is worldwide in distribution.

4.7.3 Causative agents	The anthropophilic dermatophytes *E. floccosum*, *T. mentagrophytes* var. *interdigitale* and *T. rubrum* are the most common causes of tinea pedis in Britain and North America. *T. rubrum* is the principal cause of chronic tinea pedis. *T. mentagrophytes* usually causes more inflammatory lesions.

Tinea pedis is a very widespread condition that appears to be increasing in prevalence. It often begins in late childhood or young adult life and is most common between the ages of 20 and 50. Men are more frequently affected than women.

The infection is usually acquired by walking barefoot on contaminated floors. Hyphae and arthrospores of the causal dermatophytes can survive for long periods (>12 months) in human skin scales. Excessive sweating and occlusive footwear are factors that favour the development of tinea pedis.

4.7.4 Clinical manifestations	Tinea pedis may be unilateral, but bilateral involvement is more common. Three clinical forms may be distinguished: acute or chronic interdigital infection; chronic hyperkeratotic (moccasin or dry type) infection; vesicular (inflammatory) infection. A combined clinical presentation may also occur.

Acute or chronic interdigital infection is the most common

form of tinea pedis and is characterized by itching, peeling, maceration and fissuring of the toe webs. The skin beneath the whitish build-up of debris may appear red and weeping. The cleft between the fourth and fifth toes is most often involved. A foul odour is sometimes present. The infection may spread to adjacent areas of the feet, including the toe nails. In a patient with supposed chronic tinea pedis, the absence of nail involvement makes the diagnosis of dermatophytosis questionable.

Chronic hyperkeratotic infection is characterized by areas of pink skin covered by fine white scaling. Vesicles and pustules are absent. Hyperkeratosis is usually limited to the heels, soles and lateral borders of the feet. The distribution of the infection may be patchy or involve the entire weight-bearing surface, in which case the disease is termed 'moccasin' or 'dry type' tinea pedis. The condition may be asymptomatic.

Vesicular infection is characterized by the development of vesicles, usually beginning on the sole, the instep and the interdigital clefts. The eruptions vary in size, may be isolated or coalesce into vesicles or bullae, and are initially filled with a clear fluid. After rupturing, the lesions dry, leaving a ragged ring-like border. The disease may resolve without treatment, but often recurs.

In certain parts of the world, concomitant mould, candidal and/or bacterial infection is relatively common in patients with tinea pedis. These conditions usually represent secondary infection following fissuring or maceration of a toe cleft. The secondary infection may induce inflammation and further maceration.

**4.7.5
Differential
diagnosis**

The symptoms and clinical signs of tinea pedis can be difficult to distinguish from those of a number of other infectious causes of toe web intertrigo, such as *Candida albicans* or bacterial infection. Non-infectious conditions which resemble tinea pedis include contact dermatitis, eczema, idiopathic keratoderma and psoriasis.

Candidosis most often presents with mild interdigital erosion and maceration. It sometimes occurs in patients with diabetes mellitus and is more common in hot climates. It often occurs in conjunction with a dermatophyte infection.

Other moulds which produce lesions indistinguishable from tinea pedis include *Scytalidium dimidiatum* (*Hendersonula toruloidea*) and *S. hyalinum* (see Chapter 6).

Bacterial infection tends to produce more inflammatory lesions, often with marked erosion of the skin. Erythrasma

(*Corynebacterium minutissimum* infection) is also difficult to distinguish from interdigital tinea pedis.

Laboratory tests should be performed in any patient with foot lesions of undetermined origin.

4.7.6
Essential
investigations
and their
interpretation

Direct microscopic examination of infected material should confirm a clinical diagnosis of dermatophyte infection where arthrospores and/or hyphae are seen. It is sometimes possible to distinguish *C. albicans* infection from tinea pedis by the appearance of characteristic yeast cells. Isolation of the aetiological agent in culture will permit the species of fungus involved to be determined. Media containing actidione (cycloheximide) should not be used if infection with a *Scytalidium* species is suspected.

Wood's light examination of the lesion should be performed to establish whether the patient has erythrasma. However, the coral red fluorescence, characteristic of this condition, does not exclude coexistent tinea pedis.

4.7.7
Management

Tinea pedis will often respond to topical treatment with an imidazole compound, such as clotrimazole, econazole, miconazole or sulconazole, or an allylamine such as naftifine or terbinafine. This should be applied to the toe clefts and other affected sites morning and evening for at least 2 weeks. Often 4 weeks' treatment will be required. The patient may also benefit by applying the cream to the soles to help prevent the infection from spreading. The recurrence rate following topical treatment is quite high, and chronic infection with minor scaling that persists despite treatment is not uncommon. Exacerbations of previous infection may also occur.

Mixed fungal and bacterial infections of the feet are common. For this reason, topical antifungal preparations that are effective against dermatophytosis and candidosis, and which possess some antibacterial action (such as miconazole) are recommended.

If the disease is extensive, involving the sole and dorsum of the foot, or there is acute inflammation, oral treatment with itraconazole (100 mg/d for 4 weeks) or terbinafine (250 mg/d for 2–6 weeks) should be given in addition to topical treatment. The latter should be continued for 8 weeks or longer. However, relapse is common.

Chronic tinea pedis is often associated with nail infection. Inadequate treatment of onychomycosis may result in re-infection of the feet.

Tinea pedis is a chronic condition which seldom resolves if left untreated. Exacerbations, which tend to occur in the summer, alternate with partial remissions. Nevertheless, the prognosis in general remains benign.

It is important to inform the patient of measures that may help to control or prevent the infection. Daily bathing of the feet, followed by careful drying of the toes and interdigital spaces, is important. The patient should also be advised to avoid heavy occlusive footwear, which may increase sweating, and to wear soft absorbent socks.

Once the clinical signs and symptoms have cleared, use of an anti-fungal foot powder on the feet and inside footwear may prevent reinfection.

4.8 Tinea manuum

4.8.1 Definition

The term tinea manuum is used to refer to dermatophyte infections of one or both hands.

4.8.2 Geographical distribution

The condition is worldwide in distribution.

4.8.3 Causative agents

The anthropophilic dermatophytes *E. floccosum*, *T. mentagrophytes* var. *interdigitale* and *T. rubrum* are the most common causes of tinea manuum. Less commonly, the condition is caused by zoophilic dermatophytes, such as *M. canis* and *T. verrucosum*, or geophilic dermatophytes, such as *M. gypseum*.

Hand infection may be acquired as a result of contact with another person, with an animal, or with soil, either through direct contact, or via a contaminated object such as a towel or gardening tool. Autoinoculation from another site of infection can also occur. Manual work, profuse sweating and existing inflammatory conditions, such as contact eczema, are predisposing factors.

4.8.4 Clinical manifestations

Tinea manuum is usually unilateral, the right hand being more commonly affected.

Lesions on the dorsum of the hand or in the interdigital spaces appear similar to those of tinea corporis. They have a distinct margin and central clearing may occur.

Two clinical forms of palmar infection may be distinguished: the dyshidrotic or eczematoid form; and the hyperkeratotic form. In the former condition, periods of partial remission intervene between successive exacerbations. In contrast, the hyperkeratotic form is chronic and spontaneous healing does not occur. It is not unusual for one form to turn into the other.

The dyshidrotic form of tinea manuum is characterized in the acute stage by vesicles which tend to appear in an annular or segmental pattern. These are localized to the edges of the hand, to the lateral and palmar aspects of the fingers, or to the palm itself where the vesicles are rather larger, tense, often single, and contain a clear viscous fluid. Removal of the top of the vesicles exposes a pinkish-red weeping surface with fine scaling margins. Pruritus, formication and burning are common symptoms.

The hyperkeratotic form of tinea manuum is a subacute or chronic condition. It begins as a succession of adjacent vesicles which desquamate. This results in a reddened scaling lesion which is round or irregular in outline and enclosed by a thick white squamous margin from which extensions run straight towards the centre. Once the chronic stage is reached, the disease involves most or all of the palm and fingers. The dry hyperkeratosis, with underlying erythema, readily causes fissuring in the palmar creases. The hand has a mealy appearance because of the furfuraceous scales that remain adherent to the horny layer. This is thickened and black in the creases.

**4.8.5
Differential
diagnosis**

Tinea manuum must be distinguished from other forms of dyshidrosis. This condition, whatever its origin, is usually bilateral or even symmetrical. In its typical form, clear vesicles are grouped on the lateral and volar aspects of the fingers as well as on the palm. There is little or no inflammation of the base. Dyshidrotic eczema is usually bilateral, but mycological examination is often required to distinguish it and other conditions (such as psoriasis, whether pustular or not) from tinea manuum.

**4.8.6
Essential
investigations
and their
interpretation**

Direct microscopic examination of infected material, such as vesicle tops and contents and skin scales, should reveal the branching hyphae characteristic of a dermatophyte infection. Isolation of the aetiological agent in culture will permit the species of fungus involved to be determined.

**4.8.7
Management**

Local treatment with a topical imidazole, such as clotrimazole, econazole, miconazole or sulconazole, will often suffice to clear tinea manuum.

In chronic cases that fail to respond to local treatment,

oral griseofulvin (500–1000 mg/d) or itraconazole (100 mg/d for 4 weeks) should be prescribed.

4.9 Tinea unguium

4.9.1 Definition

The term tinea unguium is used to describe dermatophyte infections of the finger nails or toe nails.

4.9.2 Geographical distribution

The condition is worldwide in distribution.

4.9.3 Causative agents

Fungal infection of the nails may be caused by a number of dermatophytes as well as by a number of other moulds (see Chapter 7) and *Candida* species (see Chapter 5). The dermatophytes most commonly implicated are anthropophilic species, such as *T. mentagrophytes* var. *interdigitale* and *T. rubrum*. Their prevalence differs from one geographical region to another. Zoophilic species, such as *T. verrucosum*, are infrequently isolated and usually only from finger nails.

Tinea unguium is most prevalent between the ages of 20 and 50, but the actual incidence of the condition is difficult to assess. This is because many reports do not distinguish between dermatophytosis and other forms of onychomycosis, or between infections of the finger and toe nails.

4.9.4 Clinical manifestations

Toe nails are more commonly infected than finger nails. Tinea unguium of the toe nails is usually secondary to tinea pedis, while finger nail infection often follows tinea manuum, tinea capitis or tinea corporis. Tinea unguium may involve a single nail, more than one nail (both hands and feet), or in exceptional circumstances, all of them. The first and fifth toe nails are more frequently affected, probably because footwear causes more damage to these nails. Finger nail infections are usually unilateral.

In most cases of onychomycosis due to dermatophyte infection the lesion, which is often white or yellow in colour with irregular edges, appears first at the free distal edge of the nail. It spreads slowly and may eventually affect the entire nail, which becomes thickened, opaque, lustreless and yellow in colour. There is usually some subungual hyperkeratosis which results in the nail becoming detached from the nail bed. The nail plate may crumble, beginning at the free edge. Paronychial inflammation is absent.

**4.9.5
Differential
diagnosis**

The clinical signs of tinea unguium are often difficult to distinguish from those of a number of other infectious causes of nail damage, such as *Candida albicans*, mould or bacterial infection. Unlike dermatophytosis, candidosis of the nails (see Chapter 5) usually begins in the proximal nail plate; nail fold infection (paronychia) is also present. Mould infections of nails are described in Chapter 7. Bacterial infection, particularly when due to *Pseudomonas aeruginosa*, tends to result in black discoloration of nails.

Noninfectious conditions which resemble tinea unguium include: nail dystrophies of assorted origin; subungual hyperkeratosis such as is found in onychogryposis; nail changes due to chronic eczema and psoriasis.

**4.9.6
Essential
investigations
and their
interpretation**

Laboratory confirmation of a clinical diagnosis of tinea unguium should be obtained whenever possible before oral treatment is commenced. This is important for several reasons: because of the long periods of treatment that are usually required; because of the high costs of such treatment; and because of the potential side effects of such treatment.

It is not uncommon to obtain negative results from culture of nail specimens from patients with dermatophytosis. One reason for this is that good specimens are often difficult to obtain. If possible, the specimen should exclude the distal edge of the nail. The affected nail should be cut as far back as possible and through its entire thickness, taking care to obtain as much crumbly material as possible. Subungual debris is seldom useful and, if included, should be submitted as a separate specimen.

The following methods of obtaining nail specimens are recommended. If distal subungual lesions are present, use a curette, spatula, or nail elevator to obtain debris from under the distal edge of the nail. If there is superficial nail plate involvement, take thin superficial scrapings with a curette, scalpel or nail elevator. If there is proximal subungual involvement, a nail drill or scalpel may be used to obtain debris. Material should be taken from any discoloured, dsytrophic or brittle parts of the nail.

Direct microscopic examination of infected nail material should confirm a clinical diagnosis of fungal infection. It is sometimes possible to distinguish *C. albicans* infection, or infection due to moulds such as *Scopulariopsis brevicaulis* from tinea unguium.

Isolation of the aetiological agent in culture will permit the species of dermatophyte involved to be determined. It is essential to inform the laboratory if nail material is suspected of being infected with moulds, so that duplicate plates with and without actidione (cycloheximide) can be inoculated.

4.9.7
Management

Tinea unguium is a difficult condition to treat. Using oral griseofulvin, up to 90% of finger nail infections can be cured in 4–8 months, but toe nail infections may take 9–12 months or longer and at least 20–40% of affected nails fail to respond. Long-term relapse rates, 12 months after griseofulvin treatment, are high; between 40% and 70% for toe nails but somewhat lower for finger nails.

The usual adult dose of oral griseofulvin is 500 mg/d given after food, but this can be increased to 1000 mg/d. Not less than 10 mg/kg should be given. The duration of treatment will depend on the clinical response, but 12 months may be required for toe nail infections. Mycological tests should be repeated at intervals after starting treatment and again before discontinuing the drug.

Encouraging results have been obtained with oral terbinafine (250 mg/d) in patients with dermatophytosis of the finger nails or toe nails. Much shorter treatment periods are required than with griseofulvin: 3 months or less is often sufficient to cure a finger nail infection. Toe nails may require treatment for 6 months or longer.

Oral itraconazole (200 mg/d) has been used to treat nail infections that failed to respond to griseofulvin, but the drug is not licensed for this indication. At least 3 months' treatment is required for success with finger nails and 5 months for toe nails.

Topical antifungals, such as amorolfine or tioconazole, may be applied to affected finger nails or toe nails. Treatment must be continued without interruption until cure is obtained. Usually, at least 6 months' treatment is required for success with finger nails and 9–12 months for toe nails.

5   Superficial Candidosis

5.1   Definition

The term candidosis (candidiasis) is used to refer to infections due to organisms belonging to the genus *Candida*. These opportunist pathogens can cause acute or chronic deep-seated infection in debilitated individuals (see Chapter 11), but are more often seen causing mucosal, cutaneous or nail infection.

5.2   Geographical distribution

These conditions are worldwide in distribution.

5.3   The causal organisms and their habitat

Although *Candida albicans* is the most important cause of superficial forms of candidosis, at least eight other members of the genus are recognized as human pathogens. Most of these organisms are dimorphic, growing as round or oval yeast cells or as pseudomycelium. *C. albicans* can also form true mycelium, but *C. glabrata* (which used to be classified as *Torulopsis glabrata*) never forms mycelium or pseudomycelium.

These organisms can be isolated from the mouth and intestinal tract of a substantial proportion (30–50%) of the normal population and from the genital tract of up to 20% of normal women. *C. albicans* accounts for 60–80% of isolations from the mouth, and 80–90% from the genital tract. However, it is seldom recovered from the skin of normal individuals, being much less prevalent than other members of the genus, such as *C. parapsilosis* and *C. guilliermondii*. Unlike *C. albicans*, which is seldom found in the environment, *C. tropicalis*, *C. parapsilosis* and a number of other pathogenic members of this large genus can sometimes be recovered from plants or soil.

In most patients, infection with *C. albicans* is derived from the individual's own endogenous reservoir in the mouth and intestinal tract. In some cases, however, the infection is acquired from another person. For instance, neonatal oral candidosis is more common in infants born of mothers with vaginal candidosis, which suggests that infection occurs when the infant takes in some of the vaginal contents during parturition. The hands of mothers are another potential source of infection in infants.

Individuals colonized with *C. albicans* possess numerous complicated and often interdependent mechanisms to prevent the organism from establishing an infection. Efficient protection is believed to involve both humoral and cell-mediated immunological mechanisms. Nonspecific mechanisms are also important, but it is well recognized that the contribution of particular elements to protection against mucosal, cutaneous and deep-seated forms of candidosis is different. Even trivial impairments of these mechanisms are often sufficient to allow *C. albicans*, the most pathogenic member of the genus, to establish a cutaneous or mucosal infection. More serious impairment of the host can lead to life-threatening deep-seated infection, often with less pathogenic organisms, such as *C. parapsilosis*.

5.4   Clinical manifestations

5.4.1
Oral candidosis

Oral candidosis can be classified into a number of distinct clinical forms: acute pseudomembranous candidosis; acute atrophic candidosis; chronic atrophic candidosis; chronic hyperplastic candidosis; and chronic mucocutaneous candidosis (see Section 5.4.6).

Acute pseudomembranous candidosis (thrush) tends to occur in infants and in old age. It is otherwise unusual unless the individual is suffering from a serious underlying condition, such as HIV infection or leukaemia. It can occur in patients using aerosolized corticosteroids for asthma or other forms of chronic obstructive lung disease.

Acute pseudomembranous candidosis presents as white raised lesions that appear on the buccal mucosa, gums or tongue. If left untreated, these can develop to form confluent plaques. The lesions may spread to involve the throat, giving rise to serious dysphagia. The lesions are often painless, although mucosal erosion and ulceration may occur.

It is important to distinguish this condition from chronic hyperplastic candidosis (oral leukoplakia). The simplest test is to determine whether the white pseudomembrane can be dislodged. If it can, leaving an eroded, erythematous, bleeding surface, then this is diagnostic for acute pseudomembranous candidosis.

Acute atrophic candidosis usually occurs as a complication of broad-spectrum antibiotic treatment. It can affect any part of the oral mucosa. If the tongue is affected, the dorsum is depapillated, shining and smooth. Tongue movement is restricted and swelling results in trauma to the lateral borders if a natural dentition is present. The mouth is often so tender that the patient finds it difficult to tolerate solid food, and consumption of hot or cold liquids causes severe pain.

Chronic atrophic candidosis (denture stomatitis) is the most common form of oral candidosis. It is usually associated with oral prostheses, occurring in up to 60% of denture wearers. The condition is asymptomatic, often being discovered only when a new prosthesis is required. The usual presenting complaint is associated angular cheilitis. Lower dentures are seldom involved. The characteristic presenting signs are chronic erythema and oedema of the portion of the palate that comes into contact with dentures.

Angular cheilitis often develops in association with other forms of oral candidosis, in particular denture stomatitis, but it may occur without signs of other oral disease. The condition is common in patients with moist, deep folds at the corners of the mouth. These angular folds are often due to a decrease in facial height due to worn dentures. Angular cheilitis can occur in non-denture wearers, including AIDS patients. The characteristic presenting signs are soreness, erythema and fissuring at the corners of the mouth.

Chronic hyperplastic candidosis (candida leukoplakia) is an important condition because the lesions can undergo malignant transformation. About 5% of all oral leukoplakias become malignant, but for candida leukoplakias the figure is 15–20%. It remains unclear whether this condition is a hyperplastic lesion superinfected with *C. albicans* or the converse.

The most common site of chronic hyperplastic candidosis is the inside surface of one or both cheeks or, less often, on the tongue. The lesion is usually asymptomatic and the condition is often associated with smoking or local trauma due to dental neglect. Lesions range from small translucent white areas to large dense opaque plaques. Lesions which contain both red erythroplakic and white leukoplakic areas must be regarded with great suspicion as malignant change is often present. In contrast to the pseudomembranous form of oral candidosis, the lesions cannot be rubbed from the surface of the buccal mucosa.

5.4.2
Vaginal
candidosis

Vaginal candidosis is a common condition, and while most patients respond well to treatment, in some the infection is intractable and chronic, or recurrent. *C. albicans* is the most important cause of vaginal candidosis, accounting for over 80% of infections. *C. glabrata* is the second most common fungus recovered from the genital tract of women with vaginitis, accounting for about 5% of infections.

The fact that a certain proportion of women harbour *C. albicans* in the genital tract without apparent symptoms or clinical signs of infection suggests that, in those women in whom symptoms or signs are present, there is some underlying host defect or precipitating factor. Although it has proved difficult to discover what host defects allow symptomatic vaginal infection with *C. albicans* to occur, the condition has been associated with a number of precipitating factors.

Vaginal candidosis is much more common in pregnant women. Moreover, infection at this time is the initiating event in a significant proportion of women with chronic or recurrent candidosis. The condition is also more common among women with diabetes mellitus, a disorder which has been implicated as a predisposing factor in other superficial forms of candidosis. Tight, insulating clothing and antibiotic treatment are among the other factors that have been recognized as predisposing to vaginal candidosis. However, aberrations of iron metabolism and oral contraception are no longer regarded as significant precipitating factors.

Most women with vaginal candidosis complain of intense vulval and vaginal pruritus and burning with or without vaginal discharge. The condition is often abrupt in onset and, in the nonpregnant woman, usually begins during the week prior to menstruation. Some nonpregnant women complain of recurrent or increasing symptoms preceding each menstrual period. Pruritus is often more intense when the patient is warm in bed, or after a bath. Dysuria and superficial dyspareunia are common.

Vulval erythema with fissuring is the most common clinical finding. This is often localized to the mucocutaneous margins of the vaginal introitus, but can spread to affect the labia majora. Perineal intertrigo with vesicular or pustular lesions may be present. Vaginitis with discharge is another common clinical finding. The classical sign of florid vaginal candidosis in the pregnant woman is the presence of thick white adherent plaques on the vulval, vaginal or cervical epithelium. This is a useful sign in the nonpregnant patient as well. Often the discharge is thick and white and contains curds, but it can be thin or even purulent. Vulvitis may be present without a concomitant vaginal infection.

Vaginal candidosis is but one of a number of causes of vulvovaginitis and vaginal discharge and must be distinguished from other conditions such as bacterial vaginosis and trichomoniasis. The clinical diagnosis of these infections is difficult and clinical suspicion must be confirmed with microbiological tests. It is also important to remember that some patients will have more than one genital infection.

5.4.3
Penile
candidosis

In men, genital candidosis usually presents as a balanitis or balanoposthitis. Patients often complain of soreness or irritation of the glans penis; less commonly there is a subpreputial discharge. Maculopapular lesions with diffuse erythema of the glans penis are often present; on occasion there is oedema and fissuring of the prepuce. Itching, scaling cutaneous lesions are sometimes found on the penis or in the groin.

Insulin-dependent diabetic men may present with an acute fulminating oedematous form of balanoposthitis with ulceration of the penis and fissuring of the prepuce. White plaques will be found on gentle retraction of the prepuce.

On occasion a male contact of a woman with vaginal candidosis will complain of soreness and itching of the glans penis soon after intercourse and lasting for 24–48 hours.

The diagnosis of candida balanitis should not be made on clinical grounds alone as there are other causes of balanitis and balanoposthitis. Specimens for mycological investigation should be taken from the coronal sulcus.

5.4.4
Cutaneous
candidosis

C. albicans is the most important cause of cutaneous candidosis. The lesions tend to occur in the folds of the skin, such as the groin and the intergluteal folds, where maceration and occlusion give rise to warm moist conditions. Lesions can also arise in small folds, such as the interdigital spaces between the fingers.

The lesions of superficial cutaneous candidosis (intertrigo) usually develop as vesicles and pustules deep in the groin and other skin folds. Friction leads to rupture of the pustules and development of erythematous lesions with an irregular margin. The main lesion is often surrounded by numerous small papulopustules, termed satellite lesions. Application of topical steroids will alter the appearance of the lesions, making them difficult to distinguish from those of dermatophytosis.

Interdigital lesions (sometimes termed erosio interdigitalis blastomycetica) arise as small fissures deep in the interdigital folds, with surrounding thickened white skin. The condition is often uncomfortable and may be painful. It is usually seen in individuals whose occupations necessitate frequent immersion of the hands in water. Interdigital candidosis is often associated with onychia and paronychia of the same hand.

In infants with the uncommon condition, congenital cutaneous candidosis, discrete vesicopustules on an erythematous base are present at birth or appear soon thereafter. The lesions usually begin on the face, neck and trunk and spread to involve the whole surface in about 24 h. This condition is thought to result from intrauterine or interpartum infection. The condition has a benign course, a desquamative phase preceding complete clearing of the lesions. In occasional patients congenital cutaneous infection can progress to deep-seated candidosis.

The precise role of *C. albicans* in the evolution of rashes on the buttocks and in the perianal region of infants, associated with wearing napkins (diapers) remains unclear. This condition should not be considered a primary candida infection as it is preceded by an irritant dermatitis.

Other cutaneous forms of candidosis include the erythematous, macronodular lesions seen in about 10% of neutropenic patients with disseminated deep candidosis, and the purulent follicular and nodular cutaneous lesions seen in heroin abusers (see Chapter 11).

5.4.5 Onychia and paronychia

Nail and nail fold infections with candida tend to occur in individuals whose occupations necessitate repeated immersion of the hands in water. The fingers affected tend to be those of the dominant hand; fourth and fifth fingers are involved less often than thumbs and middle fingers. The condition is more common in women than men. Infection of the toe nails is much less frequent. Among the various species implicated, *C. albicans* and *C. parapsilosis* are the most common.

In almost all cases the disease starts with involvement of the nail fold. The nail wall becomes swollen, erythematous and painful. The disease usually starts in the proximal nail fold, but the lateral margins are sometimes the first site to be affected. The lesion spreads round the nail, but tends to remain more pronounced in the region of the nail matrix. The swelling is often sufficient to lift the wall from the underlying nail plate.

Nail plate involvement often follows, infection usually

commencing in the proximal section. White, yellow, green or black marks appear in the proximal and lateral portions of the nail and then in the distal parts. The nail becomes more opaque, and transverse or longitudinal furrowing or pitting occurs. The nail becomes friable and may become detached from its bed. Unlike dermatophyte infections, pressure on and movement of the nail is painful.

Bacterial superinfection is a common problem. In this situation it is often difficult, if not impossible, to decide which was the initial organism.

Candida nail disease must be distinguished from a number of other nail disorders. Unlike dermatophytosis, which often begins in the distal and lateral parts of the nail, candida infection usually starts in the proximal portion. In cases of doubt the diagnosis can be established by mycological examination.

**5.4.6
Chronic
mucocutaneous
candidosis**

The term chronic mucocutaneous candidosis is used to describe a group of uncommon conditions in which individuals with congenital immunological or endocrinological disorders develop persistent or recurrent mucosal, cutaneous or nail infections with *C. albicans*. The disease often appears within the first 3 years of life. The mouth is the first site to be involved, but lesions then appear on the scalp, trunk, hands and feet. The nails and sometimes the whole of the fingertips are affected.

Chronic mucocutaneous candidosis is common in individuals with disorders in which T-lymphocyte activation is impaired or production of T-cell factors needed for macrophage activation is subnormal. These defects are often specific to *C. albicans*, but some patients have more profound defects that involve the T-cell-mediated response to other organisms as well. Patients with chronic mucocutaneous candidosis seldom develop deep-seated infection, despite their widespread or generalized cutaneous or mucosal lesions.

Chronic mucocutaneous candidosis can be classified into a number of distinct clinical forms: chronic oral candidosis; chronic mucocutaneous candidosis with endocrinopathy; chronic localized mucocutaneous candidosis (candida granuloma); chronic diffuse mucocutaneous candidosis; and chronic candidosis with thymoma.

In chronic oral candidosis, the patients have chronic pseudomembranous infection of the mouth. Angular cheilitis is often present. The major symptom is chronic pain and soreness in the mouth. This group of patients does not have cutaneous or nail infection. Occasional patients develop oesophagitis. There is no recognized genetic inheritance pattern, but the condition is more common in females than males.

The chronic candidosis with endocrinopathy syndrome typically begins in childhood. The mouth is nearly always affected and lesions may also appear on the hands, feet and nails. One or more endocrine disorders develop after the onset of the candida infection. The most common is hypoparathyroidism, but hypoadrenalism, hypothyroidism and diabetes mellitus also occur. In most cases, the first endocrinopathies appear within a few months. However, because endocrine dysfunction may be delayed until adulthood, children with chronic mucocutaneous candidosis should undergo assessment of endocrine function at annual intervals.

Chronic localized mucocutaneous candidosis (candida granuloma) has no recognized inheritance pattern, but usually begins in childhood. Patients with this syndrome may or may not have endocrinopathies. The typically disfiguring lesions are markedly hyperkeratotic, granulomatous and vegetating, affecting the mucous membranes, skin, and nails.

Chronic diffuse candidosis is a common form of mucocutaneous candidosis. It usually begins in childhood, but has no associated endocrine disorders. The erythematous lesions are widespread over the skin, nails and mucous membranes, often with serpiginous borders and little hyperkeratosis. Two genetic inheritance patterns are recognized: an autosomal recessive form and an autosomal dominant form.

Chronic candidosis with thymoma is a rare condition which does not develop until after the third decade of life. Like chronic diffuse candidosis, this adult-onset form is characterized by recalcitrant infections of mucous membranes, nails and skin, without associated endocrine disorders. In addition to candidosis, the patients often have other disorders associated with thymomas, such as myasthena gravis, myositis, aplastic anaemia, neutropenia and hypogammaglobulinaemia. Patients presenting with adult-onset chronic mucocutaneous candidosis should be evaluated at intervals for an associated thymoma.

5.5 Superficial candidosis in special hosts

Over 80% of HIV-positive individuals develop oral candidosis at some time during their illness. The development of this condition is often the initial clinical manifestation in asymptomatic individuals and is one of several clinical signs that have been associated with an increased likelihood of progression to AIDS. Both pseudomembranous and atrophic forms of oral candidosis occur, but the latter, which is often asymptomatic, usually occurs earlier and is often missed. The lesions of the pseudomembranous form are persistent and often spread to affect all parts of the mouth. Angular cheilitis has been reported in up to 20% of HIV-positive individuals.

5.6   **Essential investigations and their interpretation**

The clinical manifestations of oral candidosis are often characteristic, but can be confused with other disorders. For this reason, the diagnosis should be confirmed by demonstration of the various morphological forms of the fungus in smears prepared from swabs or scrapings of lesions and its isolation in culture. As *Candida albicans* is a normal commensal in the mouth, its isolation alone cannot be considered diagnostic of infection. Swabs should be moistened with sterile water or saline prior to taking the specimen, or sent to the laboratory in transport medium.

The diagnosis of vaginal candidosis depends on a combination of typical symptoms and signs and the demonstration of the fungus in smears or its isolation in culture. The latter is much more sensitive and reliable (about 90%) than the former (about 40%). Swabs should be taken from discharge in the vagina and from the lateral vaginal wall, and sent to the laboratory in transport medium.

Intertriginous candidosis is often difficult to diagnose if the lesions are other than typical in appearance. Isolation of *C. albicans* from swabs or scrapings is of dubious significance, because the organism is a frequent colonizer of a range of cutaneous lesions. Microscopic demonstration of the organism in scrapings of lesions is much more significant.

The diagnosis of nail fold infections rests in part on the characteristic clinical appearance. However, microscopic examination and culture is needed to confirm the diagnosis. Material can be taken from the swollen periungual nail wall, or from under the nail fold using a disposable microbiological loop or moistened swab. Pus can be obtained from under the nail fold by applying light pressure. Microscopic demonstration or isolation of the fungus from nail can be difficult with proximal lesions, but material from a distal or lateral lesion, together with subungual debris, will often reveal the diagnosis.

5.7 Management

5.7.1 Oral candidosis

In most infants with oral candidosis, the lesions clear within 2 weeks of commencing topical treatment. The condition can be trated with nystatin oral suspension (100 000 units/ml) or amphotericin oral suspension (100 mg/ml) which should be dropped into the mouth after each feed or at 4–6-h intervals.

Older children and adults with the acute pseudomembranous form of oral candidosis can be treated with nystatin or amphotericin oral suspension (1 ml at 6-h intervals for about 2–3 weeks). Miconazole oral gel may also be used. The usual adult dose is 10 ml oral gel (250 mg miconazole) at 6-h intervals. In children aged over 6, the recommended dose is 5 ml at 6-h intervals; in children aged 2–6, 5 ml at 12-h intervals, and in children under 2, 2.5 ml at 12-h intervals. It is essential that any medication should be retained in the mouth for as long as possible. Treatment should be continued for at least 48 h after all symptoms have disappeared.

Chronic atrophic candidosis is treated with good denture hygiene and topical antifungal agents. When the condition is resolved, a new prosthesis is usually required. Angular cheilitis will respond well to a topical antifungal preparation containing steroids.

In HIV-positive individuals with oral candidosis the relapse rate with topical antifungal treatment is high, and now that safe oral agents are available, these are to be preferred. This applies in particular to the treatment of pseudomembranous candidosis where there is a risk of oesophageal infection. Oral ketoconazole is not well absorbed in AIDS patients because of reduced gastric acid production. Other potential complications are liver damage (albeit rare) and interference with adrenal hormone metabolism when given in high doses. As with ketoconazole, serum concentrations of itraconazole are reduced when gastric acid production is impaired, and also during concomitant treatment with rifampicin or phenytoin. However, a dose of 200 mg/d for 4 weeks has proved effective. Oral fluconazole, at a dose of 50–100 mg/d for 1–2 weeks, has been found to be safe and perhaps more effective than ketoconazole in controlling oropharyngeal candidosis in AIDS patients.

Up to 50% of AIDS patients with oral candidosis will relapse within 1 month of the successful completion of treatment. Indefinite maintenance treatment with fluconazole (150 mg weekly) has sometimes been adopted, although intermittent dosing (depending on symptoms) has been advocated to prevent the emergence of azole-resistant strains of *C. albicans*.

5.7.2 Vaginal candidosis

Most patients with vaginal candidosis respond to topical treatment with nystatin or an imidazole, such as clotrimazole or miconazole. Nystatin gives an average mycological cure rate of 75–80%, which is lower than that achieved with the azoles.

If a patient is to be treated with nystatin, one or two vaginal tablets (100 000 units each) should be inserted high in the vagina at bedtime for 14 consecutive nights, regardless of an intervening menstrual period. If vulvitis is a problem, nystatin cream should also be applied for 2 weeks.

Four imidazole derivatives are available in a number of topical formulations for the treatment of vaginal candidosis: clotrimazole, miconazole, econazole and isconazole. These drugs give higher cure rates than nystatin (85–90%) with shorter courses of treatment, and with all there is a similar low relapse rate. These drugs are safe and side effects after topical application are uncommon. Treatment regimens range in duration from one to six nights, but treatment courses of less than six nights should be reserved for first episodes.

Itraconazole and fluconazole have been licensed for the short-term oral treatment of vaginal candidosis. These drugs are no more effective than the topical preparations, but are more expensive. Fluconazole is given as a single 150 mg dose and itraconazole is given as two 200 mg doses 8 h apart with food. Side effects are infrequent and limited to mild gastrointestinal upset.

Women with recurrent vaginal candidosis (more than three episodes within 12 months) present a difficult management problem. These patients often suffer from depression and develop psychosexual problems. It is important to make a correct diagnosis and to ensure that the patient avoids potential precipitating factors, although these may not be obvious. Physical examination and mycological investigation are essential and, if possible, should be performed when the patient is symptomatic, but has had no treatment. It is thought that in a substantial proportion of women, symptomatic recurrence results from vaginal relapse following inadequate treatment of a previous episode.

The treatment options include the use of intermittent prophylactic regimens with single-dose topical or oral antifungals to prevent symptomatic episodes. Local treatment with the single-dose (500 mg) formulation of clotrimazole at 2-week intervals has been shown to permit suppression of symptoms even if mycological cure is not achieved. Intermittent single-dose (150 mg) oral treatment with fluconazole is also effective. After symptoms have been suppressed for 3–6 months, regular treatment can be discontinued to allow patient reassessment. In many women there is no relapse to the previous pattern to frequent recurrence.

Administration of nonabsorbable oral nystatin, given to reduce intestinal colonization with *C. albicans*, has no effect on vaginal recurrence rates. Neither topical nor oral treatment of the male partner affects the relapse rate.

5.7.3
Penile
candidosis

Genital candidosis in men should be treated with local applications of an antifungal cream. Nystatin should be applied morning and evening for at least 2 weeks. Clotrimazole, miconazole or econazole creams should be applied morning and evening for at least 1 week. The female contacts should also be investigated.

5.7.4
Cutaneous
candidosis

Topical antifungal drugs should be used to treat uncomplicated intertriginous candidosis. Treatment with combination preparations containing topical steroids, such as clotrimazole or miconazole with hydrocortisone, will bring about rapid relief of the pruritus associated with this infection. If intertriginous candidosis is associated with an underlying condition, such as diabetes mellitus, control of the underlying problem is essential.

Napkin dermatitis with associated candida infection may be treated with combination topical preparations. Although more potent steroids can be used in the short term, it is advisable to use preparations containing hydrocortisone if possible. Mothers of affected infants should be advised of the basic irritant cause of the problem.

The prognosis in congenital cutaneous candidosis is good, and spontaneous cure often occurs after several weeks. The use of topical antifungals, such as nystatin or an imidazole, will hasten the cure.

5.7.5
Onychia and
paronychia

Management of nail infections is difficult, requiring prolonged oral or topical treatment and/or evulsion of the nail.
Affected nails should be bathed for 10–15 min daily in
0.01% phenyl-mercuric borate. Topical antifungals, such as
1% imidazole cream or lotion, should then be applied.
Clinical and mycological cure can often be achieved in
2–3 months, provided the factors predisposing to infection,
and sources of potential reinfection, can be corrected or
eradicated.

If topical treatment is unsuccessful, oral treatment with
itraconazole (200–400 mg/d) should be attempted. If the
infection persists, surgical or nontraumatic removal of the
nail should be considered.

5.7.6
Chronic
mucocutaneous
candidosis

In most patients, oral and cutaneous lesions will respond to
short courses of antifungal treatment. Much longer courses
of treatment are needed to clear nail infections. However,
the improvement is often transient and the infection will recur
unless the underlying immunological defect is corrected.

Oral treatment with ketoconazole has led to a marked
improvement in the condition of a substantial number of
patients, but protracted treatment is required to sustain
remission, and this can lead to the development of drug
resistance. In the near future, itraconazole and fluconazole
may become available for this condition. Although these
drugs may be no more effective than ketoconazole, they will
probably be safer for long-term use.

6   Other Cutaneous Fungal Infections

6.1   Pityriasis versicolor

**6.1.1
Definition**

Pityriasis versicolor (tinea versicolor) is a common, usually mild but often recurrent skin infection which manifests as patches of fine scaling and hypopigmentation or hyperpigmentation.

**6.1.2
Geographical
distribution**

The disease is worldwide in distribution but is most prevalent in tropical climates, where up to 50% of the population may be affected. In temperate regions it accounts for up to 4% of all dermatological disorders.

**6.1.3
The causal
organisms and
their habitat**

The aetiological agent of pityriasis versicolor is a dimorphic fungus named *Malassezia furfur*. On direct microscopic examination of material from skin lesions this organism appears as clusters of yeast cells together with short, stout curved filaments which are seldom branched.

If scrapings from pityriasis versicolor lesions are cultured on a suitable medium, it is usual to isolate two morphologically distinct lipophilic yeasts named *Pityrosporum orbiculare* (with globose cells) and *P. ovale* (with oval cells). However, these yeasts can also be recovered from normal skin, casting doubt on their aetiological role in pityriasis versicolor.

Although it is not possible to be certain, it does seem probable that *P. orbiculare* is the causative agent of pityriasis versicolor: it is recovered from lesions of this condition in over 90% of cases; the round or oval budding cells found in culture are identical to those seen on microscopic examination of scrapings from lesions; ultrastructural and antigenic similarities between *P. orbiculare* and *M. furfur* have been identified.

However, *P. orbiculare* has been isolated not only from normal skin but also from sebhorrhoeic skin, while *P. ovale* is a ubiquitous skin organism. Moreover, cultures of lesions invariably yield large bizarre yeast cells which belong to neither *P. orbiculare* nor *P. ovale*. Nor have single spore cultures from scales of pityriasis versicolor ever yielded colonies of Pityrosporum. Therefore it is conceivable that the rapid growth of Pityrosporum in culture inhibits the growth of another hypothetical fungus (also necessarily lipophilic) which is the true cause of pityriasis versicolor.

For the time being, and until more is known about this problem, it is therefore better to regard the role of Pityrosporum as uncertain, and to continue to refer to the agent causing pityriasis versicolor as *Malassezia furfur*.

The precise conditions which lead to the development of pityriasis versicolor have not been defined, but host and environmental factors appear to be important. The lesions have a predilection for sites well supplied with sebaceous glands, such as the chest, back and upper arms, and are never found on the soles or palms, which are devoid of these glands. The disease occurs in all age groups, but is less common in children and the aged, whose skin surface contains fewer lipids. Instances where noncohabiting members of the same family have developed the disease suggest a genetic predisposition.

The condition is most common during the hot summer months.

Human-to-human transmission is possible, either through direct contact or via contaminated clothing or bedding. In practice, however, spread of infection between partners is uncommon, and no cases of occupational infection among medical or nursing staff have been described.

6.1.4
Clinical
manifestations

Pityriasis versicolor is a disfiguring but otherwise harmless condition. The characteristic lesions consist of patches of fine brown scaling, particularly on the upper trunk, neck and upper arms. Lesions may also appear on the face, the ears, behind the ears, the scalp, the arms and legs, the abdomen or the groin. Widespread infection can occur.

In light-skinned subjects, the affected skin may appear darker than normal. Initially, the lesions are light pink in colour but grow darker, turning a pale brown shade. In dark-skinned or tanned individuals, the affected skin loses colour and becomes depigmented (pityriasis versicolor alba).

The same patient may have lesions of different shades, the colours depending on the thickness of the scales, the severity of the infection and the inflammatory reaction of the dermis, and in particular the amount of exposure to sunlight, which may vary from one lesion to another.

On examination of lesions under Wood's light a greenish, golden yellow or pinkish luminescence can be seen in 90% of cases, permitting the extent of the disease to be judged even in those sites where the lesions are poorly or not at all visible.

There are no reports of complications of this disease.

6.1.5 Differential diagnosis

In tanned patients, the disease must be distinguished from erythrasma, which is localized to the inguinal, axillary and inframammary folds, and to the webs of the toes. It is not unusual for the two diseases to occur in the same patient.

The depigmented form is most frequently confused with pityriasis alba, which is not uncommon among children and young women. It usually occurs in late summer or autumn, and is often localized to the face, the outside of the arms, and the shoulders. The eruptions are less well demarcated and the scaling is coarser; they look grey and fluoresce under Wood's light. Vitiligo is generally easy to recognize with its very well-defined and completely depigmented areas; it generally involves the face, the extremities and genital region.

6.1.6 Essential investigations and their interpretation

MICROSCOPY

Microscopic examination of the cleared scales is sufficient to permit the diagnosis of pityriasis versicolor if round or oval budding spores, together with stout, curved fragmented hyphae which are seldom branched, are seen.

CULTURE

Culture is seldom required for diagnosis. Scrapings from a lesion should be inoculated on to the surface of a Sabouraud's agar plate which is then overlaid with a layer of olive oil and incubated at 27–30°C. Small, cream-yellow heaped colonies will develop within 1 week.

Microscopic examination of a direct mount from the culture will reveal numerous yeast cells 3.0–5.0 μm in diameter with a thick refractile cell wall. These are designated *P. orbiculare*. There are also smaller yeasts 1.0–2.5 μm in diameter or elongated or bottle-like in form and sometimes budding. These are designated *P. ovale*. Round cells with germ tubes (hyphae) of variable length can also be seen, along with larger yeast cells, 7.0–8.0 μm in diameter, of a round shape and sometimes budding, which cannot be assigned to either the orbiculare or the ovale type.

6.1.7 Management

Treatment of pityriasis versicolor consists of the application of various topical agents, particularly selenium sulphide or an imidazole derivative such as clotrimazole, miconazole or sulconazole.

Selenium sulphide 2.5% suspension should be applied to the lesions and left on overnight at weekly intervals on no more than four occasions.

Topical imidazoles should be applied morning and evening for 4–6 weeks. Cure has been achieved if negative results are obtained on two occasions in both clinical (Wood's light) and mycological tests.

Pityriasis versicolor tends to be a difficult disease to clear completely, and any one of these preparations may need to be reused at intervals to ensure that the infection is completely eradicated.

Oral treatment with itraconazole is also effective in this condition. The usual dose is 200 mg/d for 1 week.

Griseofulvin and terbinafine are ineffective.

If left untreated, pityriasis versicolor may persist indefinitely. More than 50% of cases respond to treatment, but the organism may persist in sites where the topical agents have not been properly applied, such as the scalp or body folds, and relapse may occur. Although reinfection cannot be ruled out, it has seldom been observed.

6.2 Piedra

The term piedra refers to two uncommon diseases characterized by nodular lesions situated on and along the hair shafts. These two disorders are distinguished according to the colour and consistency of the nodules and the aetiological agent. White piedra is less common than black piedra. Acquisition of piedra does not seem to be related to personal hygiene or exposure to infected persons, nor does white piedra of the pubic hair seem to spread by sexual contact.

6.3 White piedra

6.3.1 Definition

The term white piedra is used to refer to a fungal infection of hair of the scalp and facial hair and sometimes pubis, characterized by soft greyish-white nodules of variable consistency arranged in rows on the hair shafts, to which they are adherent.

6.3.2 Geographical distribution

White piedra is found worldwide, but is most common in tropical or subtropical regions.

6.3.3
The causal
organism and
its habitat

The disease is caused by *Trichosporon beigelii*, a filamentous yeast that forms arthrospores and blastospores, hyphae, and pseudohyphae (see also Chapter 27). It penetrates between the cells of the cuticle but does not invade the hair shaft itself. *T. beigelii* has a widespread natural distribution, primarily in soil and decaying plant matter.

The disease is most common in young adults. Although there are reports of familial infection, the contagiousness of the disease is slight. Certain cosmetics or lotions may serve as a vehicle of infection. Diabetic glycosuria would appear to be a predisposing factor in the development of pubic lesions.

6.3.4
Clinical
manifestations

The presence of irregular, soft, white or light brown nodules, 1.0–1.5 mm in length, along the hairs is characteristic of white piedra. The nodules are firmly adherent to the hairs, particularly the midshafts, sometimes forming actual sheaths that taper towards each end of the hair. Occasionally the nodules do not adhere firmly and can be readily detached. The hair shaft looks normal in the areas not covered with nodules. No broken hairs are seen. The surrounding skin is unaffected.

The infection is localized to the hairs of the scalp, beard and moustache; very much less commonly the hairs of the genital, perineal and scrotal areas are affected. On the scalp only localized areas are generally involved; in other hairy skin regions, however, there is a more widespread distribution of nodules. The skin surface is intact and the nodular lesions are mainly located on the distal half of the hair shaft.

6.3.5
Differential
diagnosis

White piedra can be confused with pediculosis, trichomycosis axillaris or hair casts.

6.3.6
Essential
investigations
and their
interpretation

MICROSCOPY

The nodules, when squashed in potassium hydroxide, show that the fungus penetrates between the cells of the cuticle, which it raises by means of septate hyphae between 2 and 4 μm in diameter. The hyphae disintegrate into rectangular, oval or round arthrospores, which cluster together and sometimes show budding.

CULTURE

Hairs should be inoculated on to the surface of Sabouraud's agar plates and incubated at 25–30°C. Identifiable cream, whitish or yellowish colonies will appear within 2–3 days.

These consist of hyaline mycelium, which is septate and fragmented into rectangular, oval or round arthrospores; numerous blastospores are also present.

6.3.7
Management

Shaving, if possible, or clipping hairs of affected areas is the simplest method of treatment. Because the infection sometimes recurs after the area has been clipped or shaved, twice-daily topical treatment is recommended. Clotrimazole or miconazole cream are suitable.

6.4

Black piedra

6.4.1
Definition

The term black piedra is used to refer to a hair disease characterized by the appearance of dark brown or black nodules which adhere to the distal portion of the scalp hairs.

6.4.2
Geographical distribution

Black piedra has been reported mostly from tropical regions of Central and South America and occasionally from hot, humid parts of Asia and Africa. In South America Hispanics, Amerindians and Afro-Americans are known to be affected.

6.4.3
The causal organism and its habitat

The disease is caused by *Piedraia hortae*, a saprophytic mould, which penetrates the cuticle, but does not invade the hair shaft itself.

The natural habitat of *P. hortae* other than mammalian hair is not known. Certain hygienic habits, such as the application of plant oils to the scalp hair, seem to predispose to the condition.

Black piedra affects young adults of both sexes with a slight predominance among men. There are reports of epidemics in families and communities. The infection is spread by the common use of combs, hairbrushes or utensils used for washing the hair.

6.4.4
Clinical manifestations

The disease is localized to the scalp and appears in the form of small nodules 1–2 mm in diameter which adhere to the hair, particularly to its distal third. Affected hairs generally show from four to eight, or more, dark nodular concretions. These are spindle-shaped or conical, very hard, blackish-brown in colour, and enclose the hair in a sheath of variable density. At the edge there is a fringe of radial filaments, which are often split at their ends. The underlying skin surface is unaltered. If a fine-tooth comb is run through the infected hair, there is a kind of grating, as if there were sand in it. The hair shaft does not show any changes between the nodules. No broken hairs are seen.

6.4.5
Differential
diagnosis

Black piedra can be confused with trichorrhexis nodosa and trichonodosis, but diagnosis is usually straightforward and is based on the demonstration of blackish-brown nodules on the distal third of the hairs. These nodules cannot be confused with those of white piedra, which are light-coloured and soft, nor with those of lepothrix, which are found in the axillary and perigenital areas, nor with the nits of pediculosis. Mycological examination will always confirm the diagnosis.

6.4.6
Essential
investigations
and their
interpretation

MICROSCOPY
Microscopical examination of affected hairs will reveal the nodules partially or completely surrounding the hair shaft. These can be seen to consist of packed, pigmented mycelial filaments. They are often fragmented to form arthrospores and arranged in more or less clearly defined threads; at the edge, the filaments are roundish.

CULTURE
Hair fragments should be implanted in the usual media and incubated at room temperature. Identifiable brown or black colonies appear after 2–3 weeks. They have an irregular surface, a more or less convoluted appearance and the margins are irregular. Microscopy of a direct mount from the colony reveals dark hyphae, of a brown or orange colour, irregular in shape, septate and branched, with frayed-out ends.

6.4.7
Treatment

Therapy is the same as for white piedra.

6.5

Tinea nigra

6.5.1
Definition

The term tinea nigra is used to refer to a rare, chronic superficial mycosis with a predilection for the palms and soles which is due to *Exophiala werneckii*, a dematiaceous (brown) mould.

6.5.2
Geographical
distribution

The disease is encountered in Southeast Asia, Africa and in the tropical and subtropical regions of the American continent. Sporadic cases have been reported from North America, Britain and France.

6.5.3
The causal
organism and
its habitat

Exophiala werneckii (*Cladosporium werneckii*) is a sapro-phytic mould found in the soil and on decomposing plant matter.

Tinea nigra most commonly occurs in young adults: a light complexion and hyperhidrosis of the palm are predis-posing factors.

Although familial infections have been reported, the condition does not appear to be transmissible between humans.

6.5.4
Clinical
manifestations

Tinea nigra is usually restricted to the palm of one hand. In rare cases the fingers, soles of the feet, toes, wrists, chest, neck and, exceptionally, the face may also be affected.

The skin lesion consists of one and sometimes several flat, slate-coloured, brown or black patches with irregular pigmentation, usually without scaling, and with a well-defined and sometimes slightly raised rim. The patches are very small at first, then later expand and become confluent, forming polycyclic or irregularly contoured lesions.

Erythema and other signs of inflammation are absent. The disease is asymptomatic and may remain undiagnosed for a long time.

6.5.5
Differential
diagnosis

Tinea nigra must be differentiated from naevus, lentigo maligna, a superficially expanding melanoma, stains (typi-cally silver nitrate), a pigmented, fixed erythema, post-inflammatory pigmentation, and secondary syphilis with black discoloration.

6.5.6
Essential
investigations
and their
interpretation

MICROSCOPY
Microscopy of scales taken from the margin of the lesions will reveal a dense mycelium, consisting of hyaline, light-coloured, yellowish or dark brown hyphae, which are branched and have thick-walled septa; the segments are often irregular.

CULTURE
Scrapings should be inoculated on to Sabouraud's agar plates and incubated at 23–28°C. Identifiable black colonies of *Exophiala werneckii* should appear within 1 week.

6.5.7
Treatment

Many methods of treatment have proved effective. Benzoic acid compound (Whitfield) ointment or an imidazole de-rivative should be applied morning and evening. Treat-ment must be continued for at least 3 weeks to avoid recur-rence.

6.6

Hendersonula toruloidea and *Scytalidium hyalinum* infection

These moulds have been isolated from skin infections of the hand and foot, as well as from nail infections (see Chapter 7), in patients from the tropics and subtropics. Skin infections may be severe, resembling chronic dermatophytosis, or very mild and almost symptomless.

Microscopic examination of infected material shows chains of hyaline arthrospores which may be difficult to distinguish from those of a dermatophyte.

Both fungi are resistant to many of the antifungal drugs so far tested. It has become widely recognized that these infections are extremely recalcitrant to treatment, and at the present time no consistently effective therapy can be recommended. In vitro sensitivity to terbinafine has been reported and the drug may be useful clinically.

7   Mould Infections of Nails

7.1

Definition

The term onychomycosis is used to describe infection of the nails due to fungi. Nail infections due to dermatophyte fungi and *Candida* species have been described in Chapters 4 and 5. This chapter deals with infections caused by other, less common fungi.

7.2

Geographical distribution

The disease is worldwide in distribution.

7.3

The causal organisms and their habitat

Various filamentous fungi other than dermatophytes (see Chapter 4) have been isolated from abnormal nails. Often these are casual, transient contaminants and direct microscopic examination of nail clippings and scrapings is negative. However, certain moulds are capable of causing nail infection and when this is so it is important that their significance is recognized.

Scopulariopsis brevicaulis, a ubiquitous soil fungus, is the most common cause of nondermatophyte nail infection. It is capable of attacking healthy nails and not merely ones with preexisting damage. Apart from Scopulariopsis the following moulds have also been identified as agents causing mycosis of the nails: *Aspergillus* species, *Alternaria* species, *Acremonium* species, *Fusarium* species, *Scytalidium dimidiatum* (*Hendersonula toruloidea*) and *S. hyalinum*.

Scytalidium dimidiatum and *S. hyalinum* have been isolated from nail infections in patients from the tropics and subtropics. Mould infections of nails have been reported in all age groups, but are most prevalent in persons over 50 years of age. Men are more commonly affected than women.

The incidence of the condition is difficult to assess from published work, but *S. brevicaulis* may account for about 3% of cases of onychomycosis. The absolute number of onychomycoses due to opportunistic fungi is small even though these fungi abound in the environment. Unlike dermatophytosis, these infections are not contagious.

7.4
Clinical manifestations

The toe nails, especially the big toe, are more frequently affected than the finger nails. The disease process usually begins along the free edge of the nail or at the lateral margins, generally with a small whitish patch, which steadily spreads. The nail gradually loses its transparency, becomes lustreless and thickens because of the friable material accumulating on the distal part of the nail bed. The surface of the nail plate becomes irregular and streaked; small pits appear. The colour of the nail also changes; it is whitish at first but then turns yellowish, greenish, brownish or blackish. The whole of the nail may become friable, being reduced to a thin residual lamella, or even become detached from the nail bed. There is nothing very specific about the appearance of these lesions.

7.5
Differential diagnosis

Mould infections of nails have no specific clinical features. For this reason mycological and histological examinations should be performed on any patient with nail lesions of undetermined origin.

7.6
Essential investigations and their interpretation

Laboratory confirmation of a clinical diagnosis of onychomycosis must be obtained before treatment is commenced.

Methods for collecting nail specimens are as detailed in Chapter 4.

Isolation of a mould is not a sufficient reason for ascribing a pathogenic role to it without further investigation. Moulds are ubiquitous and their aetiological role must be critically assessed whenever they are isolated from nail material.

The fungus must be seen on direct microscopic examination and the mould must be isolated in pure culture without the simulataneous appearance of a dermatophyte. It is sometimes possible to distinguish infections with *S. brevicaulis* from tinea unguium on microscopic examination: the characteristic, roughened thick-walled oval spores of this mould are often present in infected nails.

If an opportunistic fungus has been found on mycological investigation, the relationship between it and the nail plate can be determined with the aid of histological sections.

7.7
Management

Mould infections of nails seldom respond to antifungal

therapy. Treatment must be carried out in two phases: chemical dissolution or surgical removal of the parasitized nail followed by application of antifungal preparations. After avulsion of the affected nails 0.02% phenylmercuric borate solution or 1% potassium permanganate solution should be applied for 5–6 days. Then, when the nail bed is no longer tender, an antifungal agent active against moulds, such as an imidazole derivative, should be applied. Treatment should be continued for 8–12 months until the nails have regrown. Mycological tests should be performed at 6–8-week intervals.

The course is chronic and without treatment the infection may last years or even indefinitely. With treatment the prognosis is good, the damage being purely aesthetic.

8   Keratomycosis

8.1

Definition

The term keratomycosis (mycotic keratitis) is used to describe fungal infection of the cornea. This often follows the traumatic implantation of spores into the corneal epithelium, or their inadvertent introduction during surgical procedures, such as corneal transplantation. This infection is difficult to treat and can cause severe visual impairment or blindness.

8.2

Geographical distribution

The condition is worldwide in distribution, but is more common in the tropics. In temperate climates it is most common in rural districts.

8.3

The causal organisms and their habitat

More than 60 different fungi have been reported to cause corneal infection. Most are widespread in the environment, being found in soil, dust and decomposing plant matter. Their spores are often found in the outside air. Many of these saprophytic organisms are also common culture contaminants.

Members of the genus *Aspergillus* (in particular *A. fumigatus* and *A. flavus*) are the most common cause of keratomycosis in the Indian subcontinent, but species of *Fusarium* (in particular *F. solani*) are predominant in many other tropical and subtropical regions. Other causes of keratomycosis include *Acremonium* species, *Curvularia* species and *Penicillium* species.

Keratomycosis is most common in men, particularly those with an outdoor occupation. It usually follows some form of trauma involving plant or animal matter or other materials. The traumatizing agent itself may harbour fungal spores which are thus implanted into the cornea, or the injuring agent may cause a superficial abrasion that exposes the cornea to infection.

Many patients with keratomycosis have received topical corticosteroid or antibacterial antibiotic treatment for ocular disease, and this is an important predisposing factor.

8.4 Clinical manifestations

The clinical manifestations of keratomycosis are predictable and similar regardless of the organism involved. The initial symptoms include increasing pain, ocular redness, photophobia and blurred vision.

Examination of the affected eye should be carried out using a slit lamp. The usual clinical finding is a raised corneal ulcer with a white, ragged border. Around and beneath the ulcer is a dense infiltrate extending deep into the corneal stroma. Although the lesion has a radiating margin, the lesion is well defined. Discrete satellite lesions often develop. Involvement of the anterior chamber occurs, leading to formation of a sterile hypopyon. If left untreated, the infection will spread into the anterior chamber and result in corneal perforation and loss of the eye. Enucleation is usually required because of pain.

8.5 Essential investigations and their interpretation

Although the clinical picture is distinctive, the diagnosis of keratomycosis requires the demonstration of fungal elements on microscopic examination of smears prepared from corneal scrapings, together with the isolation and identification of the aetiological agent and the elimination of other causes for the disease.

Because the aetiological agents of keratomycosis are common contaminants of the corneal surface, isolation alone is inadequate for making a diagnosis. Nor is a superficial corneal surface specimen adequate. The organisms are often difficult to find, being located deep inside the corneal stroma, rather than on the surface.

Specimens should be taken using a platinum spatula to scrape corneal fragments from the margins and base of the ulcer. The scrapings should then be smeared on a clean glass slide and examined with a potassium hydroxide wet mount or a Gram's stain. Scrapings should also be inoculated on to plates or tubes of Sabouraud's agar supplemented with an antibacterial antibiotic, such as chloramphenicol. This is best done in the clinic. The plates should then be incubated at 25–30°C (rather than 37°C) for at least 2 weeks before being discarded as negative. The colonies of most aetiological agents of keratomycosis appear within 3–5 days. Isolation of a fungus is more convincing if multiple colonies are obtained on a plate, or if the same organism is recovered on more than one occasion.

Aspiration of a hypopyon is not recommended because it is not without risk and the fluid is usually sterile.

8.6 Management

The management of keratomycosis entails removal of infected tissue, discontinuation of corticosteroids, and topical or oral treatment with an antifungal drug.

Topical treatment with econazole (10–20 mg/ml) or miconazole (10 mg/ml) is sometimes successful. Both are applied at a rate of one drop at 15–30 min intervals. Treatment may need to be continued for 6–8 weeks or longer.

Other drugs that can be prepared for topical application include natamycin and amphotericin. Natamycin suspension (50 mg/ml in sterile water) is applied at a rate of one drop at 1–3-hour intervals. Amphotericin suspension (1–5 mg/ml in sterile water) should be applied at a rate of one or two drops per hour and at 2–3-hour intervals at night. Both these drugs have limitations: the penetration of natamycin is poor and amphotericin is toxic to the corneal epithelium.

Subconjunctival injections of amphotericin (0.5 ml of 0.125 mg/ml solution in sterile water) or of miconazole (5 mg/d) have been given but their effectiveness is uncertain.

Oral administration of ketoconazole (400 mg/d) has benefited some patients, but itraconazole (200 mg/d) has proved more successful.

Surgical intervention is often helpful in the management of keratomycosis. Superficial debridement will improve the penetration of topical antifungal drugs. Superficial or lamellar keratectomy may be effective if the lesion is small and localized, and particularly if it is located in the peripheral cornea. Penetrating keratoplasty is an effective method of eliminating infected corneal tissue since the entire thickness of the cornea is removed.

Infections with *Fusarium* species often result in rapid corneal sloughing and marked visual loss, and are difficult to treat. Aspergillus infections are less difficult to manage with antifungal drugs, but the larger the ulcer and the deeper the hypopyon, the greater the likelihood of loss of vision. Even with intensive antifungal treatment, progression to corneal perforation, scleral suppuration or anterior chamber infection can occur. Corneal scarring with consequent reduction in vision is a frequent complication, even with successful treatment.

9   Otomycosis

9.1   **Definition**
The term otomycosis is used to describe mould or yeast infection of the external auditory canal.

9.2   **Geographical distribution**
The condition is worldwide in distribution.

9.3   **The causal organisms and their habitat**
Otomycosis is most commonly caused by *Candida* species, particularly *C. albicans* and *C. tropicalis*, and *Aspergillus* species, particularly *A. fumigatus*, *A. niger*, *A. nidulans* and *A. flavus*. Other agents that have been implicated include ubiquitous saprophytic moulds, such as *Absidia* species, *Acremonium* species, *Penicillium* species, *Pseudallescheria boydii*, *Rhizopus* species and *Scopulariopsis brevicaulis*.

Otomycosis occurs in adults of all ages and of both sexes; children are less commonly affected. In temperate climates it is most commonly seen during the summer months.

Otomycosis is not a contagious condition.

Otomycosis often develops in individuals with preexisting bacterial otitis externa, eczema or seborrhoeic dermatitis of the external auditory canal. These diseases are often of long standing and have usually been treated with topical agents and corticosteroids, factors well recognized as predisposing to fungal infection.

9.4   **Clinical manifestations**
Because there are no specific symptoms, otomycosis may be confused with any form of otitis externa.

The patient usually complains of prickling, itching and burning. Two forms of otomycosis, the acute and chronic forms, are recognized.

Acute otomycosis is of abrupt onset, has a marked inflammatory character, manifested by reddening, oedema and a thick, whitish, or colourless discharge that may be foul-smelling or odourless. There may be severe ear ache. Otoscopic examination reveals whitish patches with a surface resembling felt or wet blotting paper, covered with brown, green or black dots; or whitish or greenish-brown deposits;

or total or partial obstruction of the external auditory canal by a more or less dense membranous or cotton-wool-like mass.

Chronic otomycosis causes itching and a moderate, yellowish odourless discharge. In rare cases the patient complains of burning. Otoscopic examination reveals: an appearance like wet blotting paper; exudative otitis externa, accompanied by scaling and yellowish crusts, under which there is a hyperemized and oozing integument; myringitis granulosa, in which the eardrum is covered with small, flat, pink-coloured, striped and hard granulations with ill-defined margins and one or more perforations.

The course of otomycosis is frequently complicated by the simultaneous presence of bacterial otitis externa that either preceded the fungal infection or supervened later. Eczematization of the external auditory canal and the pinna is not uncommon: it may be of bacterial origin or drum-induced.

There is frequently an impairment of hearing; it is generally mild, invariably involves conduction deafness and is usually reversible.

Perforation of the eardrum resulting in otitis media or mastoiditis is uncommon.

9.5 Differential diagnosis

The clinical diagnosis of otomycosis is difficult, although resistance to locally applied antibiotics and corticosteroids and the onset of a hearing impairment are strongly suggestive of fungal infection.

The diagnosis can be established with confidence only by mycological investigations.

9.6 Essential investigations and their interpretation

Material for mycological investigation should be obtained from the scaly or matted deposits blocking the external auditory canal. Microscopic examination will reveal branching hyphae, yeast cells with or without pseudohyphae, and also aspergillus sporing heads.

Isolation of the aetiological agent in culture will enable the species of the fungus involved to be identified.

9.7 Management

Topical nystatin suspension (100 000 units/ml), or ointment (100 000 units/g) or gel (200 000 units/g) should be applied morning and evening for 2–3 weeks. Imidazole creams such as econazole nitrate also give excellent results.

The course is chronic with acute episodes, especially in summer, and intermittent remissions. With antifungal treatment the prognosis is good.

10   Aspergillosis

10.1   Definition

The term aspergillosis is used to refer to infections due to moulds belonging to the genus *Aspergillus*. In its most serious form there is widespread growth of the fungus in the lungs and dissemination to other organs often follows. This condition occurs in compromised individuals and is fatal if left untreated. Human disease can also result from noninfectious mechanisms: inhalation of spores of these ubiquitous organisms can cause allergic symptoms in both atopic and non-atopic individuals.

10.2   Geographical distribution

These conditions are worldwide in distribution.

10.3   The causal organisms and their habitat

Most human infections are caused by *Aspergillus fumigatus*, but *A. flavus*, *A. nidulans*, *A. niger* and *A. terreus* have also been implicated. These moulds are widespread in the environment. They are common soil inhabitants and are also found in large numbers in dust and decomposing organic matter. Their spores are often found in the outside air.

Most infections follow inhalation of aspergillus spores that have been released into the air and the lungs or paranasal sinuses are the most common sites of damage. Less commonly, infection follows traumatic implantation of spores as in keratomycosis (see Chapter 8), or inadvertent inoculation as in endocarditis.

Nosocomial outbreaks of aspergillosis have become a well-recognized complication of construction work in or near hospital wards in which neutropenic patients are housed. In several reported outbreaks, building works adjacent to the unit in which the patients were accommodated led to contamination of the air. In other outbreaks, the ventilation system for the unit drew contaminated air from neighbouring building sites, or otherwise became contaminated.

10.4   Clinical manifestations

Inhalation of aspergillus spores can give rise to a number of different clinical forms of aspergillosis, depending on the immunological status of the host. In non-compromised individuals, aspergillus can act as a potent allergen or cause localized infection of the lungs or sinuses.

In neutropenic patients, there is widespread growth of the fungus in the lungs and dissemination to other organs often follows. This condition is usually fatal, even if diagnosed during life and treated. It must, however, be emphasized that with early diagnosis and treatment, a small but significant number of patients are cured.

10.4.1 Allergic aspergillosis

This is an uncommon condition, most often seen in atopic individuals who develop bronchial allergic reactions (asthma) following inhalation of aspergillus spores. Mucus plugs then form in the bronchi, leading to atelectasis. The illness may be mild, but it is an episodic condition and can often progress to bronchiectasis and fibrosis.

It is thought to result from type I and III, and perhaps type IV immunological reactions to antigens released from the fungus colonizing the bronchial tree.

The most frequent symptoms include fever, intractable asthma, productive cough, malaise and weight loss. Expectoration of brown eosinophilic mucus plugs containing aspergillus mycelium is common.

The radiographic findings range from small, fleeting, unilateral or bilateral infiltrates with ill-defined margins (often in the upper lobes) and hilar or paratracheal lymph node enlargement, to chronic consolidation and lobar contractions.

10.4.2 Fungus ball of the lung

Fungus ball (aspergilloma) formation usually occurs in patients with residual lung cavities following tuberculosis, sarcoidosis, bronchiectasis, pneumoconiosis or ankylosing spondylitis. Haemoptysis is the only serious complication. Fungus balls are usually located in the upper lobes. Less frequently they occur in the apical segments of the lower lobes. Spontaneous lysis has been reported to occur in up to 10% of cases.

Patients are often asymptomatic, but may present with chronic cough, malaise and weight loss. Haemoptysis is the most common symptom, occurring in 50–80% of cases, and can, on occasion, be massive and life-threatening.

Chest radiographs will reveal a characteristic oval or round mass with a radiolucent halo or crescent of air over the superior aspect. The mass can often be shown to move as the patient changes position. Computerized tomography (CT) scans will help to delineate the lesion.

10.4.3
Acute invasive
aspergillosis of
the lung

This form of aspergillosis occurs in immunosuppressed individuals and may be fatal, even if diagnosed during life and treated. Those at risk include neutropenic patients with haematological malignancies, transplant recipients, and children with chronic granulomatous disease. There is widespread growth of the fungus in the lung tissue resulting in haemorrhagic infarction. Haematogenous dissemination to other organs often follows.

The most common presentation in the neutropenic patient is an unremitting fever (higher than 38°C) that fails to respond to broad-spectrum antibacterial treatment. Pleuritic chest pain is not unusual. Cough may be present, but sputum production is usually minimal. Haemoptysis is uncommon.

The radiological findings are nonspecific, but the earliest lesions are single or multiple nodules. These usually progress to diffuse bilateral consolidation, or cavitation, or large wedge-shaped peripheral lesions, representing haemorrhagic infarction. The latter suggest aspergillosis and their detection is sufficient justification for treatment. In 10% of patients with proven aspergillosis, the chest radiograph has been normal within a week of death.

CT scans will often reveal nodular lesions in patients with normal chest radiographs.

Expectoration of necrotic tissue from an infarcted lesion can leave behind what looks like a fungus ball of the lung. However, this should not be confused with the classical benign condition seen in the nonimmunocompromised patient.

Haematogenous dissemination of infection from the lungs to the brain, gastrointestinal tract and other organs occurs in up to 30% of patients.

10.4.4
Chronic
necrotizing
aspergillosis of
the lung

This condition usually occurs in middle-aged or older men with chronic or previously treated lung disease such as tuberculosis. Pleural spread has been reported, but dissemination beyond the lung does not occur.

The most frequent symptoms include fever, productive cough, malaise and weight loss, often lasting for months before diagnosis. The radiographic findings include a chronic progressive infiltrate representing parenchymal necrosis involving the upper lobes, or superior segment of the lower lobes. Cavitation is common and about 50% of patients develop single or multiple fungus balls.

**10.4.5
Infection of the
paranasal
sinuses**

Two different forms of sinusitis due to *Aspergillus* species: have been recognized. Acute sinusitis is a life-threatening condition encountered in immunosuppressed patients. The clinical presentation is similar to that of rhinocerebral mucormycosis (see Chapter 13). The presenting symptoms include fever, nasal discharge, headache and facial pain. Necrotic lesions develop on the hard palate or nasal turbinate, and disfiguring destruction of facial tissue may occur. The infection can spread into the orbit and brain, causing thrombosis and infarction.

Paranasal aspergillus granuloma formation is a slowly progressive condition. It is most common in the tropics, where *A. flavus* is the most prevalent cause, although cases have been reported from temperate climates. Affected individuals usually complain of long-standing symptoms of nasal obstruction and headache suggesting chronic sinusitis, but are otherwise normal. Patients present with unilateral facial pain and headache, or with facial swelling and proptosis. The swelling is firm but not usually tender. In the later stages of this condition, upward spread of the fibrosing paranasal granuloma results in focal cerebral or orbital infection.

The typical radiological finding is a dense filling defect within the maxillary or ethmoid sinuses with erosion of the surrounding bone. This can be confirmed by CT or magnetic resonance (MR) scanning.

A third form of aspergillus sinusitis, termed allergic fungal sinusitis, has recently been described.

**10.4.6
Central nervous
system
aspergillosis**

It is much more common for cerebral aspergillosis to occur following haematogenous dissemination of infection from the lungs than for it to result from direct spread from the nasal sinuses. The brain is involved in about 10% of cases of disseminated aspergillosis, but cerebral infection is seldom diagnosed during life.

The symptoms of cerebral aspergillosis are gradual in onset. Confusion, behavioural alterations and reduced consciousness in a neutropenic patient should suggest the diagnosis. Multiple brain lesions with infarction due to cerebral arterial thrombosis often result in focal neurological signs, fits and raised CSF pressure.

The CSF findings are normal in 50% of cases. In the remainder, the protein concentration may be raised, but the glucose concentration is usually normal. On occasion, a marked pleocytosis is seen. It is most unusual to recover the fungus from CSF.

CT scans are often helpful in locating the lesions, but the findings are nonspecific.

Meningitis is a most unusual manifestation of CNS aspergillosis.

10.4.7
Ocular
aspergillosis

Three forms of ocular infection with aspergillus have been recognized. The traumatic introduction of the fungus into the eye may result in a corneal ulcer that can progress to perforation (see Chapter 8).

Endophthalmitis is an uncommon condition, but it has been described in drug abusers, in patients with endocarditis, and in organ transplant recipients. It can arise following ocular trauma or haematogenous spread of the fungus. The latter is more usual in immunocompromised patients. The symptoms include ocular pain and impaired vision.

Orbital aspergillosis can develop as an extension from infection of the paranasal sinuses. The presenting symptoms include orbital pain, proptosis and loss of vision. In 25% of cases the infection spreads into the brain and causes death.

10.4.8
Endocarditis
and myocarditis

Aspergillus endocarditis tends to occur in patients undergoing open heart operations, although it has also been described as a complication of parenteral nutrition and drug addiction. The aortic and mitral valves are the most frequent sites of infection. It often gives rise to large friable vegetations and large emboli are common.

The symptoms and clinical signs are similar to those of bacterial endocarditis, with prolonged fever, and abnormal heart murmurs. More specific diagnostic signs include large friable vegetations. Emboli that obstruct major arteries, particularly those of the brain, occur in about 80% of cases.

Myocardial infection with abscess formation or mural vegetations may occur as a result of haematogenous dissemination. Myocarditis has been reported in about 15% of patients dying with disseminated aspergillosis. It can result in nonspecific ECG abnormalities or congestive heart failure.

10.4.9
Osteomyelitis

Aspergillus osteomyelitis is an uncommon condition, but children with chronic granulocytic disease seem to be at particular risk. In these children, spread from an adjacent lung lesion is usual and the ribs and spine are the most common sites of aspergillus infection. In adults, the spine is also the most common site of infection, but haematogenous spread of the fungus may be more common. Paraplegia can occur.

The symptoms include fever and recurrent back pain. The radiological findings are nonspecific, but vertebral involvement can lead to demonstrable destruction of several vertebral bodies with collapse and loss of the intervening disc space. Joint involvement is rare.

Many patients with aspergillus osteomyelitis also have surrounding soft-tissue involvement, with pleural disease and paraspinal abscesses.

**10.4.10
Cutaneous
aspergillosis**

Two different forms of cutaneous aspergillosis have been reported in immunosuppressed patients. Cutaneous lesions may arise at catheter insertion sites and act as the source of a subsequent disseminated infection. The lesions begin as erythematous to violaceous, oedematous, indurated plaques that evolve into necrotic ulcers covered with a black eschar.

In about 5% of patients with invasive aspergillosis, haematogenous spread of infection gives rise to cutaneous lesions. These may be single or multiple, well-circumscribed, maculopapular lesions that become pustular. They evolve into ulcers with distinct borders covered with a black eschar. The lesions enlarge and may become confluent.

**10.4.11
Other forms of
aspergillosis**

Gastrointestinal tract infection has been detected in 40–50% of patients dying with disseminated infection. The oesophagus is the most frequent site of involvement, but intestinal ulcers also occur and these often result in bleeding or perforation.

Hepatic and/or splenic infection has been seen in up to 30% of patients with disseminated aspergillosis. The symptoms include liver tenderness, abdominal pain and jaundice, but many patients are asymptomatic. CT scans will reveal numerous, small radiolucent lesions scattered throughout the liver. Modest elevations in alkaline phosphatase or bilirubin concentrations can often be detected.

Renal infections occur in 30% of patients dying with disseminated aspergillosis. Symptoms are uncommon and renal function is seldom impaired.

10.5

Essential investigations and their interpretation

Establishing the diagnosis of aspergillosis in a compromised patient is difficult because the clinical presentation is nonspecific and because the fungus is seldom isolated from blood or other fluids, or from sputum. Interpretation of serological test results is also difficult because failure to detect precipitins in a compromised individual does not mean that aspergillosis is not present. Nor is the detection of circulating antigen a consistent finding in such patients.

10.5.1
Microscopy

Microscopic examination of sputum preparations is often helpful in the diagnosis of allergic aspergillosis, because abundant septate mycelium with characteristic dichotomous branching is usually seen.

Microscopic examination of sputum is seldom helpful in patients with suspected invasive aspergillosis, but examination of bronchoalveolar lavage specimens is often rewarding. Typical mycelium may also be detected in wet preparations of necrotic material from cutaneous lesions or sinus washings, but isolation of the aetiological agent in culture is essential to confirm the diagnosis.

The most reliable method for the diagnosis of acute invasive aspergillosis is the examination of stained tissue sections. The detection of nonpigmented, septate filaments which show repeated dichotomous branching is characteristic of aspergillus infection. However, other less common organisms, such as *Fusarium* species and *Pseudallescheria boydii*, appear similar. More precise identification can sometimes be achieved with immunochemical staining methods.

10.5.2
Culture

The definitive diagnosis of aspergillosis depends upon the isolation of the aetiological agent in culture. The fungus may be recovered from sputum specimens from patients with allergic aspergillosis, but cultures from patients with other forms of aspergillosis are less successful. Moreover, because *Aspergillus* species are commonly found in the air, their isolation must be interpreted with caution. Their isolation from sputum is more convincing if multiple colonies are obtained on a plate, or the same fungus is recovered on more than one occasion.

If sputum cannot be obtained from an immunocompromised patient with a lung infiltrate, alveolar lavage specimens should be obtained. Isolation of an *Aspergillus* species from such specimens is often indicative of infection, but is positive in less than 60% of cases.

Aspergillus species are seldom recovered from blood, urine or CSF specimens, although cultures of the former have been positive in occasional patients with endocarditis. More often, however, their isolation is due to contamination. It has not been established whether lysis-centrifugation is any more useful than traditional blood culture methods in the diagnosis of aspergillosis.

The diagnosis of aspergillus sinusitis is less difficult to establish than infection at other sites. The fungus can usually be isolated from sinus washings or biopsies of the necrotic lesions in the nose or palate.

10.5.3
Skin tests

Skin tests with *A. fumigatus* antigen are useful in the diagnosis of allergic aspergillosis. Patients with uncomplicated asthma due to Aspergillus give an immediate type I reaction. Those with allergic aspergillosis give an immediate type I reaction and 70% also give a delayed type III reaction.

10.5.4
Serological tests

Tests for aspergillus precipitins are often helpful in the diagnosis of the different forms of aspergillosis that occur in the noncompromised patient. Precipitins can be detected in up to 70% of patients with allergic aspergillosis and over 90% of patients with fungus balls in their lung.

The precipitin test is also useful for diagnosing chronic necrotizing aspergillosis of the lung and other invasive forms of aspergillus infection, such as endocarditis, provided the patient is not immunosuppressed.

The detection of precipitins in a neutropenic patient with unresponsive fever or a lung infiltrate is often sufficient to prompt the initiation of antifungal treatment, but it must be stressed that a positive test result is not proof of infection. Nor does a negative precipitin test result preclude the diagnosis of aspergillosis in an immunosuppressed patient, because such individuals are often incapable of mounting a detectable serological response.

Tests for the detection of circulating aspergillus antigen in blood and other host fluids offer an alternative means of diagnosing aspergillosis in the immunosuppressed patient. Low concentrations of galactomannan, a cell wall glycoprotein, have been detected in patients with invasive aspergillosis. However, aspergillus galactomannan is rapidly cleared from the circulation and frequent sampling is required for optimal detection of antigen.

A latex particle agglutination (LPA) test for aspergillus galactomannan has been marketed (Pastorex Aspergillus, Diagnostics Pasteur), but should not be relied upon as the sole method for the diagnosis of invasive aspergillosis.

10.6 Management

10.6.1 Allergic aspergillosis

Mild disease may not require treatment. Prednisone is the drug of choice because it is effective in reducing symptoms, improving chest radiographs, and abolishing positive sputum cultures. The usual dosage regimen is 1.0 mg/kg per day until radiographs are clear, then 0.5 mg/kg per day for 2 weeks. The same dose is then given at 48-h intervals for another 3–6 months, and then the dose is tapered off over another 3 months. The initial regimen should be resumed if the condition recurs. Bronchodilators and postural drainage may help to prevent mucus plugging. Treatment with antifungal drugs is not thought to be helpful.

10.6.2 Fungus ball of the lung

Surgical resection is indicated if massive or recurrent haemoptysis should occur. On occasion, segmental or wedge resection will suffice, but lobectomy is usually required to ensure complete eradication of the disease.

If surgical intervention is contraindicated, endobronchial instillation or percutaneous injection of amphotericin may be helpful. The optimum dosage has not been determined, but 10–20 mg of amphotericin in 10–20 ml distilled water instilled two or three times per week for about 6 weeks has proved successful. Larger doses (40–50 mg) have been instilled into lung cavities using percutaneous catheters.

The treatment of mild to moderate bleeding and asymptomatic patients remains controversial, but observation without intervention may be the best form of management.

10.6.3 Chronic necrotizing aspergillosis of the lung

Treatment with an antifungal drug, such as amphotericin, is often the first step in management, but surgical resection of necrotic lung and surrounding infiltrated tissue may also be required. The long-term prognosis is poor.

10.6.4 Infection of the paranasal sinuses

In some cases of paranasal aspergillus granuloma, surgical removal of infected material, with drainage and aeration, is curative. Often, however, the condition will recur, necessitating further surgical intervention. The long-term results are generally poor. Postoperative treatment with itraconazole appears promising as a means of preventing relapse. The drug should be given at a dosage of 200 mg/d for at least 6 weeks.

Neutropenic patients with acute aspergillus sinusitis require surgical debridement and treatment with amphotericin (1.0 mg/kg per day).

10.6.5 Endophthalmitis

Patients with aspergillus endophthalmitis should be treated with parenteral amphotericin (1.0 mg/kg per day). Surgical debridement and intravitreal instillation of amphotericin (two or three 5 μg doses) may also be required.

10.6.6 Endocarditis

Aspergillus endocarditis requires aggressive medical and surgical treatment. Treatment with high-dose amphotericin (1.0 mg/kg per day) alone is ineffective. Infected tissue and prostheses must be removed.

10.6.7 Osteomyelitis

Surgical debridement of necrotic tissue is important in the management of aspergillus osteomyelitis. Most patients with vertebral osteomyelitis undergo simple debridement as part of their initial diagnostic procedure. Later procedures include radical debridement with bone grafting. Both medical and surgical treatment are required if ribs are infected.

Treatment with itraconazole (400 mg/d) has proved successful in several patients with aspergillus osteomyelitis.

10.6.8 Cutaneous aspergillosis

High-dose amphotericin (1.0 mg/kg per day) is the treatment of choice. Debridement of cutaneous lesions that arise at catheter insertion sites should be delayed until the neutrophil count has recovered.

10.6.9 Acute invasive aspergillosis

The successful management of acute invasive aspergillosis in the neutropenic patient depends on the prompt initiation of antifungal treatment (within 96 h of the onset of infection). The prognosis is poor if the neutrophil count does not recover.

The drug of choice for the treatment of disseminated aspergillosis is amphotericin. There are numerous regimens for administration of this drug, but widespread agreement that in neutropenic patients it is important to give the full dose of amphotericin from the outset (see Chapter 3). High doses *must* be used (at least 1.0 mg/kg per day).

Liposomal amphotericin (AmBisome) is much better tolerated and doses as high as 3–5 mg/kg per day have been administered without significant side effects. Administration of the drug in this form has sometimes eradicated aspergillus infection in neutropenic patients, and it should be considered in patients who have failed to respond to the conventional parenteral formulation, or who have developed side effects that would otherwise necessitate discontinuation of the drug.

The optimum duration of treatment has not been established, but amphotericin should be continued at least until the neutrophil count is more than $0.5 \times 10^9/l$. Thereafter treatment should be continued until symptoms resolve and relevant radiological abnormalities (on radiographs and CT scans) disappear.

The shortcomings of current methods of diagnosis often require clinicians to proceed to amphotericin treatment without waiting for formal proof that a neutropenic patient with persistent fever ($> 72-96$ h duration), resistant to antibacterial drugs, has aspergillosis. Empirical treatment should be initiated with the usual test dose (1 mg) of amphotericin. If possible, the full therapeutic dosage level should be reached within the first 24 h of treatment.

Treatment with itraconazole (400 mg/d) has sometimes proved successful in neutropenic individuals with invasive aspergillus infection. However, absorption of the drug from the gastrointestinal tract can be a problem and blood concentrations *must* be measured at regular intervals (see Chapter 3 for a discussion of the role of prophylactic treatment with this drug). Miconazole, ketoconazole and fluconazole have no place in the treatment of aspergillus infection in the compromised patient.

Neutropenic patients who recover from aspergillosis may suffer from reactivation of the infection during subsequent periods of immunosuppression. One solution to this problem is to begin empirical treatment with amphotericin (1.0 mg/kg per day) not less than 48 h before antileukaemic treatment is commenced. The drug should then be continued until the neutrophil count has recovered.

11   Deep Candidosis

11.1

Definition

The term candidosis (candidiasis) is used to refer to infections due to organisms belonging to the genus *Candida*. In addition to causing mucosal and cutaneous infection (see Chapter 5), these opportunist pathogens can cause acute or chronic deep-seated infection in debilitated individuals. This may be confined to one organ or become widespread (disseminated candidosis).

11.2

Geographical distribution

These conditions are worldwide in distribution.

11.3

The causal organisms and their habitat

Candida albicans is the predominant cause of both superficial and deep-seated forms of candidosis, although the proportion of serious infections attributed to other members of the genus is rising. *C. tropicalis* has emerged as an important pathogen in neutropenic patients and *C. parapsilosis* infection is common in patients receiving parenteral nutrition. Other significant pathogens, such as *C. glabrata*, *C. lusitaniae* and *C. krusei*, have been noted to be resistant to certain antifungal drugs, highlighting the need for careful speciation of organisms before commencing treatment. Most members of the genus are dimorphic, growing as round or oval yeast cells or as pseudomycelium. *C. albicans* can also form true mycelium, but *C. glabrata* (which used to be classified as *Torulopsis glabrata*) never forms mycelium or pseudomycelium.

These organisms are found in the mouth and gastrointestinal tract of around 30–50% of normal individuals, but much higher isolation rates have been recorded among patients receiving medical attention.

Most cases of deep-seated candidosis occur in debilitated individuals who are predisposed to infection from their own endogenous reservoir. Unequivocal single-strain outbreaks of candidosis due to cross-infection between hospital patients have sometimes been reported.

Lethal, deep-seated forms of candidosis tend to occur in two distinct groups of patients. The first consists of individuals rendered neutropenic as the result of an underlying malignant condition or its treatment: the gastrointestinal tract is the principal source of infection in this group and the liver, spleen and lungs are often involved. Most of the second group are surgical or burns patients: these individuals are debilitated, but not neutropenic: disruption of natural anatomical barriers permits the organisms to gain access to the circulation. Patients who have had organ transplants, or operations on the heart or gastrointestinal tract, are most at risk of developing candidosis.

Administration of drugs that cause ulceration of the mouth or gastrointestinal tract is an important predisposing factor because this site is the usual source of organisms that give rise to deep-seated forms of candidosis. Broad-spectrum antibiotics are regarded as predisposing factors because their administration often has a profound effect on the microbial population of the gastrointestinal tract and can lead to proliferation of *C. albicans* in the intestinal contents. Insertion of vascular catheters for drug administration or parenteral nutrition disrupts anatomical barriers against infection and is an additional factor predisposing individuals to candidosis.

11.4 Clinical manifestations

11.4.1 Oesophagitis

This condition often develops in AIDS patients or following treatment for cancer. It tends to occur in patients with oral candidosis, but must be distinguished from cytomegalovirus (CMV) and herpes simplex virus (HSV) oesophagitis, which can give rise to similar symptoms and clinical and radiological findings. It often occurs in conjunction with viral oesophagitis.

The principal symptoms are painful dysphagia with substernal chest pain and burning. Nausea and vomiting may occur.

Barium contrast radiographs often reveal irregular ragged mucosal margins, ulcers, large filling defects or oedematous mucosal folds. Endoscopic examination is required to confirm the diagnosis. The characteristic finding is white plaques with intense inflammation. This method has established a diagnosis of oesophageal candidosis in up to 25% of patients with normal oesophagrams.

Mediastinitis may follow oesophageal perforation and stenosis can be a late complication.

**11.4.2
Gastrointestinal
candidosis**

This condition is often asymptomatic and is seldom diagnosed during life. Mucosal ulcerations are the most common lesions. Perforation can lead to disseminated deep-seated infection.

**11.4.3
Pulmonary
candidosis**

This condition is seldom diagnosed during life. It can arise following haematogenous dissemination of organisms or as a result of endobronchial inoculation of the lung. In newborn infants, infection often follows aspiration of organisms from the mouth.

The clinical and radiological presentation is nonspecific. Haematogenous dissemination gives rise to diffuse nodular infiltrates affecting both lungs. Endobronchial inoculation results in a local or diffuse bronchopneumonia.

**11.4.4
Central nervous
system
candidosis**

This is uncommon. Meningitis is the most frequent presentation and is apt to occur in low-birth-weight infants with deep-seated candidosis and in patients with ventriculoperitoneal shunts. If often follows an indolent course with minimal fever. Hydrocephalus can result from chronic meningitis or shunt obstruction. The diagnosis is difficult and the condition is fatal if untreated. *C. albicans* is the principal aetiological agent.

The CSF findings are varied. As in other forms of meningitis, the protein concentration may be increased, the glucose concentration may be low or normal, and a neutrophilic or lymphocytic pleocytosis may be present.

Other less common forms of CNS candidosis include brain abscess and diffuse metastatic encephalitis. These manifestations are seldom diagnosed during life. Large brain abscesses may give rise to focal neurological signs. These can be detected with CT scans. More often, however, haematogenous spread of organisms results in multiple small lesions that produce no neurological deficits.

**11.4.5
Endocarditis,
myocarditis and
pericarditis**

Infection with *C. albicans* is the most common form of fungal endocarditis. Three groups of individuals develop this condition: patients with underlying native valve disease, patients with prosthetic heart valves, and intravenous drug abusers. The aortic and mitral valves are the most frequent sites of infection, but the tricuspid valve is often involved in drug abusers. Infection with *C. tropicalis* and *C. parapsilosis* has been common in drug abusers.

In surgical patients, endocarditis tends to occur within the first 2 months after the operation. The prognosis has been poor and more than 80% of patients given antifungal treatment alone have died. Earlier and improved surgical intervention has led to more patients surviving.

The symptoms and clinical signs are similar to those of bacterial endocarditis, with prolonged fever, heart murmurs, and an enlarged spleen. More specific diagnostic signs include large vegetations, arterial obstructions and endophthalmitis.

Myocardial infection with abscess formation is a complication of endocarditis, but it may also occur as a result of haematogenous spread. It has been found in 50% of patients dying with disseminated candidosis. The diagnosis is difficult. Nonspecific ECG abnormalities are common.

Purulent pericarditis is an unusual complication of haematogenous dissemination of *C. albicans* infection. It can arise also from extension of a superficial myocardial abscess.

**11.4.6
Renal
candidosis**

It is much more common for renal candidosis to result from the haematogenous spread of organisms than for it to occur as a result of ascending infection. At least 80% of patients with disseminated candidosis develop renal infection. This often results in abscess formation. Less commonly, it results in the formation of clumps of mycelium which can obstruct the pelvis or ureters leading to hydronephrosis or anuria.

The symptoms of renal candidosis include fever, rigors, lumbar pain and abdominal pain. Oliguria and anuria are common presenting signs in infants with this infection. There are no specific radiological signs, apart from fungus balls in the renal pelvis or ureters, which appear as radiolucent, irregular filling defects.

**11.4.7
Lower urinary
tract candidosis**

This often results from the local spread of organisms from the genital or gastrointestinal tract. It is more common in women than men and tends to occur in diabetics or patients with abnormal or damaged urinary tracts. Many infections are related to an indwelling urethral catheter. The clinical presentation is varied, duration may be transient or prolonged, and the prognosis may be good or bad.

**11.4.8
Hepatic and
splenic
candidosis**

Hepatosplenic candidosis has emerged as a distinct clinical syndrome in leukaemic patients who have regained an adequate neutrophil count after remission induction treatment. Typically, the infection begins while the patient is neutropenic and presents as fever that fails to respond to antibacterial treatment. In most cases there are no discernible lesions in any organ, nor are there signs of infection in any particular organ. The neutrophil count then returns to normal, but fever persists, often associated with continuing weight loss.

The patient may complain of abdominal pain, and hepatic and/or splenic enlargement may be detected. Many patients have highly elevated serum concentrations of alkaline phosphatase, but other liver function abnormalities may be mild or absent.

The diagnosis should be suspected if CT scans reveal numerous small radiolucent lesions in the liver or spleen.

Microscopic examination of stained sections of biopsied tissue will often confirm the diagnosis, but the organism is isolated from no more than 30% of specimens. Blood cultures are negative. *C. albicans* is the principal aetiological agent, but *C. tropicalis* has sometimes been implicated.

11.4.9
Peritonitis

C. albicans peritonitis is an uncommon complication of peritoneal dialysis. It can also occur as a result of gastrointestinal perforation or contamination from a leaking intestinal anastomosis. Previous antibiotic treatment is an important predisposing factor.

The presenting symptoms include abdominal pain and tenderness, with or without nausea, vomiting or fever.

11.4.10
Intrauterine candidosis

Although symptomatic candidosis of the lower genital tract is one of the most common infections encountered in pregnant women (see Chapter 5), fetal infection is unusual. Intrauterine candidosis is believed to result from ascending infection of the maternal genital tract. In most cases, fetal infection follows contamination of the amniotic fluid. Spontaneous abortion associated with fetal candidosis has been reported in women fitted with an intrauterine contraceptive device.

Intrauterine candidosis presents as multiple small yellow-white lesions scattered over the surface of the umbilical cord. In some cases the fungus affects the fetus and in live births such infections manifest as the characteristic lesions of congenital cutaneous candidosis (see Chapter 5). Umbilical cord lesions are often associated with other lesions which are less characteristic and take the form of diffuse, generalized chorioamnionitis.

**11.4.11
Osteomyelitis,
arthritis and
myositis**

Infection of bone and joints often occurs as a result of the haematogenous dissemination of *C. albicans*. Inadvertent inoculation of organisms during corticosteroid injection or during insertion of a joint prosthesis can lead to arthritis.

Osteoarticular forms of candidosis, in particular vertebral, costochondral and sternoclavicular infections, are often seen in heroin abusers. Arthritis and osteomyelitis are late complications of the haematogenous spread of organisms in low-birth-weight infants and neutropenic patients.

In adult patients with osteomyelitis the lumbar spine is often involved. The symptoms include fever that is indolent in onset and back pain. The infection gives rise to characteristic well-defined osteolytic lesions. The symptoms of arthritis include indolent joint pain and effusion. It is unusual for more than one joint to be involved.

Muscular tenderness is often associated with disseminated *C. tropicalis* infections in neutropenic patients.

**11.4.12
Endophthalmitis**

This condition is increasing in incidence. It is an occasional complication of ocular trauma, but is more often seen following haematogenous dissemination of organisms. It is seldom encountered in neutropenic patients, but often occurs in heroin abusers.

The symptoms include blurred vision, ocular pain and floaters. Fundoscopic examination will reveal the typical yellow-white retinal exudate. This may be unilateral or bilateral and can develop into a vitreous abscess. Extension into the anterior chamber may occur.

In most cases infection results in blindness unless treated.

**11.4.13
Disseminated
candidosis**

This condition is not one disease: rather, it is a spectrum of different patterns of infection. Acute disseminated candidosis is a fulminant life-threatening infection most commonly encountered in neutropenic patients, in post-surgical patients, in burns patients, and in low-birth-weight infants. Of the postsurgical group, the patients who have had organ transplants, or operations on the heart or gastro-intestinal tract are at greatest risk. Chronic disseminated candidosis is an indolent illness which occurs in leukaemic patients recovering from antineoplastic treatment. Many patients with disseminated candidosis present with patterns of disease intermediate between those of the acute and chronic forms.

Acute disseminated candidosis should be suspected in a patient with persistent fever that fails to respond to broad-spectrum antibacterial treatment. Other useful clinical signs that suggest deep infection include macronodular cutaneous lesions (seen in about 10% of neutropenic patients), chorio-retinal lesions (seen in about 30% of non-neutropenic patients with candidaemia, but seldom seen in neutropenic patients), muscular tenderness, and pain in the spine or other bones.

Often, the first sign of chronic disseminated candidosis in a leukaemic patient is persistent fever that fails to disappear when the neutrophil count returns to normal. Other signs include abdominal pain, and an enlarged liver and/or spleen. Elevated levels of serum alkaline phosphatase are a help-ful sign. Fever may persist for months despite antifungal treatment.

11.5 Candidosis in special hosts

11.5.1 Low-birth-weight infants

Unifocal and multifocal forms of deep-seated candidosis can occur in low-birth-weight infants requiring prolonged neonatal intensive care. Meningitis occurs more frequently than in older patients and is sometimes associated with arthritis and osteomyelitis. Although uncommon, isolated renal infection also can occur and result in ureteric ob-struction and renal failure. Vascular catheters and admin-istration of broad-spectrum antibacterial drugs are important predisposing factors in neonatal renal candidosis.

11.5.2 Drug abusers

Addicts who inject heroin solutions contaminated with *C. albicans* often develop an unusual form of disseminated candidosis. This consists of a purulent follicular and nodular cutaneous infection associated with ocular and osteoarticular lesions. The symptoms include sudden onset of fever, rigors, headache and myalgia several hours after the injection of heroin. The fever lasts between 24 and 72 h and cutaneous lesions then appear in more than 90% of patients. Endoph-thalmitis develops in 40–60% of patients, occurring 1–2 weeks after the onset of fever. Osteoarticular lesions develop in 20–30% of patients, appearing 2 weeks to several months after the cutaneous lesions. Costrochondral involvement is the most frequent and characteristic finding.

11.5.3 AIDS patients

Oral infection with *C. albicans* (see Chapter 5) often spreads to the oesophagus in HIV-positive individuals. Oesophagitis can also occur without oral involvement, but this is unusual. Other localized forms of deep candidosis, such as meningitis and endophthalmitis, have been reported, but widespread disseminated infection is uncommon. In the few AIDS patients who have developed this condition, prolonged vascular catheterization has been an important predisposing factor.

11.6 Essential investigations and their interpretation

Establishing the diagnosis of deep-seated candidosis is difficult because the clinical presentation is nonspecific and because the results of microbiological and serological tests are difficult to interpret. In cases of suspected deep-seated candidosis, cultures should be made from as many sources as possible, and efforts should also be made to obtain material for microscopic examination.

11.6.1 Microscopy

The detection of typical blastospore or filamentous forms of *Candida* species in stained tissue sections is diagnostic of deep-seated candidosis.

11.6.2 Culture

Many members of the genus *Candida* are normal commensal inhabitants of the mouth and gastrointestinal tract, and their isolation from sputum or faecal specimens cannot be considered diagnostic of infection. Isolation from blood or other fluids, or from other closed sites, or from macronodular cutaneous lesions provides more reliable evidence of deep-seated infection. It is important that specimens are processed as soon as possible after collection to avoid problems of interpretation because of multiplication of organisms.

Blood culture should be performed in all cases of suspected deep-seated candidosis. However, it is not unusual for numerous attempts to be required before the organism is recovered. Blood should be drawn both through intravenous catheters and from peripheral veins. Lysis centrifugation is a more sensitive technique than culture in vented biphasic media or broth. Blood cultures are positive in no more than 50% of neutropenic patients with disseminated candidosis or 80% of patients with endocarditis.

Isolation of a *Candida* species from urine is often indicative of serious infection, provided the patient does not have an indwelling urethral catheter. In noncatheterized patients, care must be taken to ensure that vaginal or perineal infection does not lead to contamination of urine specimens. In infants, suprapubic aspiration is the best method of urine collection. Isolation of *C. tropicalis* from urine is more often indicative of disseminated candidosis than isolation of *C. albicans*. It has been suggested that counts of more than 1×10^4 cfu/ml in a noncatheterized patient should be regarded as significant, but this has never been validated. High counts in a patient with an indwelling catheter are seldom significant.

Isolation of organisms from the CSF provides reliable evidence for the diagnosis of meningitis, but often requires repeated culture of large amounts of fluid. All specimens obtained from ventricular shunts or reservoirs should be cultured for *Candida* species.

Particular care must be taken in interpreting the results of sputum culture as this material is often contaminated with organisms from the mouth. Culture of bronchial secretions (obtained through a bronchoscope) provides more reliable evidence of lung colonization or infection.

11.6.3
Serological tests

Serological tests should be attempted in all cases of suspected deep-seated candidosis, although the results must be interpreted with care. A single positive precipitin test result is not diagnostic of infection because the mannan and somatic antigens used are unable to distinguish antibodies formed during deep infection from those produced during mucosal colonization or infection. Nor does a negative precipitin test result preclude the diagnosis of deep candidosis in an immunosuppressed patient, because such individuals are often incapable of mounting a detectable serological response.

Precipitin methods are most useful when sequential specimens are tested at intervals over a period of time. High or rising precipitin titres should be regarded as suspicious.

Tests for the detection of precipitins are least helpful in immunosuppressed patients. In such cases, methods for the detection of circulating *C. albicans* antigen may be more useful. Low concentrations of mannan, a heat-stable cell wall component, have been detected in many patients with deep-seated candidosis. However, mannan is rapidly cleared from the circulation and frequent sampling is required for optimal detection of antigen. Several latex particle agglutination (LPA) tests for *C. albicans* mannan have been marketed.

Other circulating antigens that have been detected in patients with deep-seated candidosis include an undefined heat-labile glycoprotein antigen. The LPA test that was marketed for detection of this antigen (Candtec, Ramco

Laboratories) has often proved unhelpful and cannot now be recommended for routine use in the diagnosis of deep-seated candidosis.

11.7 Management

11.7.1 Oesophagitis

Oesophageal candidosis can be treated with oral ketoconazole (200–400 mg/d) or fluconazole (50–100 mg/d). Both drugs are given for 2–4 weeks, but fluconazole is much more reliably absorbed and less toxic than ketoconazole. Oral itraconazole (200 mg/d) is also effective.

If no improvement occurs, treatment should be changed to low-dose amphotericin (0.3 mg/kg per day). Patients who remain symptomatic after 2 weeks require further investigation for other causes of oesophagitis.

11.7.2 Endocarditis

In most instances, endocarditis requires both medical and surgical treatment. Infected prostheses should be removed about 1–2 weeks after treatment with amphotericin (1.0 mg/kg per day), with or without flucytosine (150 mg/kg per day), has been started. Earlier surgical intervention is indicated if there are large vegetations, signs of heart failure or dysfunction of a prosthesis.

The optimum length of treatment remains controversial, but continuation for 2–3 months has been recommended to reduce the likelihood of relapse.

11.7.3 Renal candidosis

There are three basic approaches to the management of renal candidosis: local irrigation of the renal pelvis with antifungal drugs, oral or parenteral treatment with antifungals, and surgical removal of obstructions or resection. In practice a combined approach is often required.

Amphotericin (1.0 mg/kg per day), with or without flucytosine (150 mg/kg per day), remains the drug of choice for renal candidosis. Fluconazole is excreted unchanged and in high concentrations in the urine. Its use is still under evaluation. It should be given in modified dosage to patients with impaired renal function (see Chapter 3). Miconazole, ketoconazole and itraconazole are not eliminated in the urine, and are therefore poor choices for treatment.

11.7.4 Lower urinary tract candidosis

Local instillation of an antifungal drug is reasonable in patients with indwelling urethral catheters if there are no signs of pyelonephritis, or of renal or ureteric obstruction. Intermittent instillation (200–300 ml of a 50 mg/l solution

at 6–8-h intervals) or continuous irrigation with amphotericin (50 mg/l in sterile water) for 5–7 days is often
successful. Oral fluconazole (50–100 mg/d) for 2–4 weeks
is the simplest option for cystitis in patients without indwelling catheters (provided the organism is susceptible).

11.7.5 Peritonitis

Peritonitis associated with peritoneal dialysis should be
treated with parenteral amphotericin (1.0 mg/kg per day)
(intraperitoneal administration of amphotericin often results
in the development of adhesions). The catheter should be
removed until the infection is cleared.

Peritonitis arising from perforation first requires surgical
repair. Parenteral amphotericin (1.0 mg/kg per day) is the
drug of choice for this condition. The role of fluconazole is
still under evaluation.

11.7.6 Endophthalmitis

Patients with endophthalmitis should be regarded as having
disseminated candidosis and should be treated with amphotericin (1.0 mg/kg per day) and flucytosine (150 mg/kg
per day). If the infection has spread into the vitreous humour
or anterior chamber, surgical intervention and intravitreal
instillation of amphotericin (two or three 5 μg doses) may be
required. The role of itraconazole and fluconazole is still
under evaluation.

11.7.7 Other deep sites

Meningitis should be treated with amphotericin (1.0 mg/kg
per day), although addition of flucytosine has been advocated
for neonatal infections. Infected shunts should be removed
or replaced.

Amphotericin is the drug of choice for osteoarticular
forms of candidosis. Surgical debridement of bone lesions is
not essential for cure. Arthritis has responded to parenteral
amphotericin, with no need for intra-articular injection.

11.7.8 Disseminated candidosis

The successful management of acute disseminated candidosis often depends on the prompt initiation of antifungal
treatment. Neutropenic patients with positive blood cultures should be considered to have disseminated candidosis
and treated. Non-neutropenic patients with positive blood
cultures often develop complications, such as endophthalmitis or osteomyelitis, and it is therefore prudent to treat
all individuals who have candidaemia.

The regimen of choice for acute disseminated candidosis
is the combination of amphotericin and flucytosine (provided the organism is susceptible to the latter drug). The

recommended dose of amphotericin is 1.0 mg/kg per day and that of flucytosine is 150 mg/kg per day. In patients with a life-threatening infection the full dose of amphotericin (50 mg) can be given from the outset (see Chapter 3). Flucytosine concentrations should be monitored at regular intervals. Provided it is possible, it is prudent to remove the central venous catheters of patients whose blood specimens (obtained either through the catheter or from a peripheral vein) have yielded a *Candida* species in culture.

Liposomal amphotericin (AmBisome) treatment should be considered in patients who have failed to respond to the conventional parenteral formulation, or who have developed side effects that would otherwise necessitate discontinuation of the drug.

The shortcomings of current methods of diagnosis often require clinicians to proceed to amphotericin treatment without waiting for formal proof that a neutropenic patient with persistent fever ($> 72-96$ h duration), resistant to antibacterial drugs, has a fungal infection. Empirical treatment should be initiated with the usual test dose (1 mg) of amphotericin. If possible, the full therapeutic dosage level (1.0 mg/kg per day) should be reached within the first 24 h of treatment. There is no need for gradual escalation of dosage, nor is there evidence to support the clinical prejudice that a lower dose can be used in suspected candidosis (see Chapter 3).

The role of itraconazole (400 mg/d) and fluconazole (400–800 mg/d) in the treatment of acute disseminated candidosis is still undergoing clinical evaluation (see Chapter 3 for a discussion of the role of prophylactic treatment with these drugs). Miconazole and ketoconazole are not recommended for the treatment of this infection.

The usual treatment for chronic disseminated candidosis (hepatosplenic candidosis) in leukaemic patients has been amphotericin, but the infection often persists despite the administration of this drug for periods of 6 months to total doses as high as 5 g. Liposomal amphotericin (AmBisome) has been more promising. Administration of the drug in this form at dosages of 3–5 mg/kg per day has eradicated hepatosplenic infection and permitted the resumption of antineoplastic treatment in some leukaemic patients.

Administration of oral fluconazole, at dosages of 400 mg/d or higher, has also proved successful in a small number of patients with hepatosplenic candidosis.

12   Cryptococcosis

12.1

Definition

The term cryptococcosis is used to refer to infections due to the encapsulated yeast *Cryptococcus neoformans*. This ubiquitous organism can cause disease in normal individuals, but a high proportion of human infections occur in compromised patients. Infection follows inhalation, but meningitis is the most common clinical presentation and widespread disseminated infection can also occur.

12.2

Geographical distribution

The condition is worldwide in distribution.

12.3

The causal organism and its habitat

Two varieties of *C. neoformans* are recognized: var. *neoformans* and var. *gattii*. Each of these can be divided into two serological groups, A and D, and B and C. There have been reports of human infections due to *C. albidus* and *C. laurentii*, but the significance of these isolations remains doubtful.

Human infection with *C. neoformans* var. *neoformans* is most prevalent in Europe and North America while infection with *C. neoformans* var. *gattii* usually occurs in the tropics including Africa and East Asia. However, var. *neoformans* has become the predominant cause of cryptococcosis in AIDS patients, even in Africa.

The most important natural source of *C. neoformans* var. *neoformans* is old, dried accumulations of pigeon droppings and soil contaminated with bird droppings. However, there have been no reports of focal outbreaks of cryptococcosis associated with disturbance of contaminated sites. The source of *C. neoformans* in pigeon droppings has not been identified. The pigeons do not appear to be infected.

C. neoformans var. *gattii* has never been isolated from pigeon droppings or soil. Its natural habitat has been identified as *Eucalyptus camaldulensis*, the red gum tree.

Inhalation of *C. neoformans* is believed to be the usual mode of infection in humans. The infectious particles could be small, desiccated, acapsular cells disseminated in the air from accumulations of dried bird droppings, or basidiospores of the perfect form of the fungus, *Filobasidiella neoformans*.

Host protection against *C. neoformans* infection is thought to depend on efficient T-cell-mediated immunological function. Impairment of T-cell function has been identified as a major factor predisposing individuals to more serious forms of cryptococcosis with rapid progression and dissemination. The profound T-cell defects that develop in individuals with HIV infection predispose them to disseminated cryptococcosis.

12.4 Clinical manifestations

Mild or subclinical infection of the lungs is the most common form of cryptococcosis, although it is diagnosed less frequently than meningitis because it is often transient and asymptomatic. It is more common for cryptococcosis to present as disseminated infection. The usual site of involvement is the central nervous system, but other organs can be affected.

12.4.1
Pulmonary cryptococcosis

In normal individuals this form of cryptococcosis is indolent in onset. The symptoms include cough, dull chest pain, mucoid sputum production, weight loss, mild fever, night sweats and malaise. Often there is no fever.

The radiological findings are variable. Mass lesions, with little or no hilar enlargement, are common. Diffuse infiltrates and peribronchial infiltrates are less frequent. Cavitation, pleural effusion, fibrosis and calcification are rare.

In immunocompromised patients, cryptococcal infection of the lungs tends to give rise to dissemination with meningitis.

Active infection of the lungs is found in some patients with other forms of cryptococcosis, in particular meningitis.

12.4.2
Meningo-encephalitis

Infection of the brain and meninges is the most common clinical form of cryptococcosis and the most common cause of death from that disease. It follows dissemination of the organism from the lungs. However, fewer than 30% of patients have such an infection at the time their meningo-encephalitis is diagnosed.

In nonimmunocompromised individuals the symptoms and signs are often indolent in onset. Headache is the most common presenting symptom: the pain is dull, bilateral and diffuse. Mental changes, such as drowsiness and confusion, also occur. Other symptoms include nausea, vomiting, neck stiffness, blurred vision or a blind spot. Fever is often minimal or absent until late in the course of the infection. Internal hydrocephalus is a serious complication.

About 90% of patients have abnormal CSF findings including increased pressure, raised protein concentration, lowered glucose concentration and a lymphocytic pleocytosis.

Solid CNS lesions occur in less than 5% of patients with neurological involvement. These lesions are insidious in onset and present with focal signs. CT or MR scans will reveal ring-enhancing or hyperdense lesions.

In AIDS patients, *C. neoformans* infection is often insidious in onset, with few meningeal symptoms or signs. Often the sole presenting symptom is mild headache. Less than 20% are somnolent, confused or obtunded. In some AIDS patients, however, the infection is much more abrupt in onset. Focal neurological findings are rare.

Hydrocephalus or ventricular dilatation can be detected and monitored with CT scans. Radionucleotide scans will reveal low-pressure hydrocephalus.

12.4.3
Cutaneous
cryptococcosis

Haematogenous spread of *C. neoformans* gives rise to cutaneous lesions in 10–15% of patients with disseminated cryptococcosis. These are single or multiple nodules, ulcers or abscesses. The lesions are often located on the head, but may occur on the trunk or limbs. Multiple small maculopapular cutaneous lesions resembling molluscum contagiosum have been found in AIDS patients.

Most patients with untreated cutaneous lesions will develop meningoencephalitis.

12.4.4
Osteomyelitis

Osteomyelitis occurs in 5–10% of patients with disseminated cryptococcosis. The pelvis, spine, prominences of long bones, cranial bones and ribs may be affected. Vertebral lesions are the most common site in patients with disseminated infection.

The symptoms include dull pain on movement. Radiographs reveal well-circumscribed, round osteolytic lesions without sclerosis.

12.4.5
Ocular
cryptococcosis

Ocular manifestations of cryptococcosis include papilloedema, motor palsies, scotoma and chorioretinitis. Papilloedema occurs in patients with cryptococcal meningoencephalitis as a result of raised intracranial pressure. It can lead to optic atrophy.

Chorioretinitis often precedes other manifestations of disseminated cryptococcosis.

12.4.6
Other forms of
cryptococcosis

Isolation of *C. neoformans* from the urine of patients with disseminated infection is not unusual. Occasional patients have clinical signs of pyelonephritis or prostatitis. Prostatic infection is a common cause of persistent urinary tract infection after apparently effective treatment for cryptococcal meningitis in patients with AIDS.

Other unusual sites of infection include the adrenal gland, heart, liver and spleen.

12.5

Cryptococcosis in special hosts

12.5.1
AIDS patients

Cryptococcosis is the most common life-threatening fungal infection in patients with AIDS, occurring in about 6–10% of such individuals in North America and up to 30% in Africa. Of patients with AIDS who develop cryptococcosis, over 80% have meningitis or meningoencephalitis at the time of diagnosis. However, infection of numerous other organs has been described, with the lungs, liver, skin and adrenal glands most commonly affected. Because the clinical presentation can be so nonspecific it is important to consider the diagnosis in all AIDS patients who present with a fever and to re-evaluate them at regular intervals for cryptococcal infection, even if the initial investigations are negative.

In addition to widespread dissemination, cryptococcosis in AIDS patients seldom responds well to treatment, and persistent or recurrent infection is common.

12.6

Essential investigations and their interpretation

Establishing the diagnosis of cryptococcosis is often less difficult than diagnosis of other fungal infections.

12.6.1
Microscopy

Encapsulated *C. neoformans* cells can often be detected in specimens of CSF or other host fluids or secretions mounted in Indian ink or nigrosin. However, lymphocytes in particular can be confused with the organism. In AIDS patients, *C. neoformans* cells are usually plentiful in the CSF, although the capsules are often small, making recognition difficult. Persistently positive CSF findings in patients undergoing treatment should be considered evidence of failure or relapse *only* if they are confirmed by a deterioration in the patient's clinical condition or by positive cultures.

12.6.2
Culture

The likelihood of isolating *C. neoformans* from CSF is increased if multiple specimens are taken and the centrifuged sediments of large amounts (4–8 ml) of fluid are plated out. The organism grows best at 30–35°C and it is advisable to prolong incubation of plates in suspected cases for up to 2 weeks.

C. neoformans can also be recovered from blood, sputum, urine, prostatic fluid and other specimens. Positive blood cultures have been obtained in 35–70% of AIDS patients with cryptococcosis. Lysis centrifugation has been the most sensitive method. Because of the greater load of organisms, microscopic examination and culture of other specimens is more often positive in untreated AIDS patients than in other individuals.

12.6.3
Serological tests

Antibodies to C. neoformans can often be detected in patients with early or localized infection, but are seldom found in patients with untreated meningeal or disseminated infection in whom tests for antigen are much more helpful.

The latex particle agglutination (LPA) test for C. neoformans capsular antigen is one of the most reliable methods for the diagnosis of a deep-seated fungal infection. Serum, urine and CSF specimens can be tested. The test is specific, provided that rheumatoid and other interfering factors are removed. False-negative results can occur if the organism load is low or if the organisms are not well encapsulated.

The LPA test for antigen should be performed on all CSF specimens at the time of diagnosis as well as on subsequent CSF specimens as one means of evaluating the response to treatment. Serum antigen levels are also useful in monitoring the response to treatment, provided they are used in conjunction with clinical evaluation of the patient. Their main advantage over CSF antigen levels is that blood can more easily and frequently be obtained.

The antigen test is positive in over 90% of patients with untreated meningeal infection. Much higher titres in both serum ($> 1:1\,000\,000$) and CSF ($> 1:64\,000$) have been detected in patients with AIDS. Levels of antigen in the CSF often decline with treatment, but the test may remain positive for several weeks. This is more common in patients whose initial load of organisms is high. Positive CSF antigen test results may be obtained despite failure to recover C. neoformans from the CSF. This may represent the persistent release of antigen from dead cells or slow elimination of capsular antigen from the CSF, rather than ongoing infection.

High or unchanging antigen levels during treatment

should be considered evidence of failure or relapse only if they are confirmed by a deterioration in the patient's clinical condition or by positive cultures.

Repeated negative tests for serum antigen in AIDS patients without neurological symptoms or signs makes the diagnosis improbable, but should not preclude the clinician who still suspects cryptococcal meningitis from performing a lumbar puncture. A positive serum antigen test should be followed by a CT or MR scan to exclude a cerebral mass lesion (due to toxoplasmosis) before a lumbar puncture is performed.

12.7 Management

All patients with cryptococcosis, apart from a few non-compromised individuals with infection of the lungs, require treatment.

12.7.1 Pulmonary cryptococcosis

Immunocompromised patients should be treated to prevent progression or dissemination of infection. Treatment is also required should symptoms persist for more than 3 weeks. If treatment is indicated, amphotericin (0.5–0.8 mg/kg per day) should be given over a 4–6-week period.

All patients with proven or suspected infection should be investigated for signs of disseminated cryptococcosis. In addition to full physical examination (with particular attention to CNS function, hepatic or splenic enlargements and cutaneous rashes), CSF, blood, urine and prostatic fluid should be cultured, and CSF and blood should be tested for antigen. These investigations should be repeated at intervals until the patient recovers.

12.7.2 Meningitis and disseminated infection

Patients presenting with meningoencephalitis should be investigated for signs of disseminated cryptococcosis. In addition to physical examination, blood, urine and prostatic fluid should be cultured, and CSF and blood should be tested for antigen. These investigations should be repeated at intervals until the patient recovers.

NON-AIDS PATIENTS

The regimen of choice for patients with meningeal or disseminated infection is the combination of amphotericin (0.3–0.5 mg/kg per day) and flucytosine (150 mg/kg per day). In patients with a life-threatening infection, the full dose of amphotericin (50 mg) can be given from the outset (see Chapter 3). In immunocompromised patients the combination regimen should be given for at least 6 weeks. In noncompromised individuals it may be effective when given for 4 weeks. Flucytosine concentrations should be monitored at regular intervals.

If there is significant deterioration in the patient's condition after treatment is initiated, or if there is no clinical improvement after 3 weeks of treatment, the dose of amphotericin should be increased to 0.6–1.0 mg/kg per day. If the patient is receiving corticosteroids their dosage should be reduced. A ventriculoperitoneal shunt should be inserted if symptomatic hydrocephalus is present. If the response is still slow, intrathecal treatment should be considered.

If amphotericin is given on its own, it should be administered in a higher dose (0.8–1.0 mg/kg per day) than that used in the combination regimen. At least 10 weeks treatment is often required.

Itraconazole and fluconazole are less toxic than amphotericin, but the role of these drugs in the treatment of cryptococcosis in non-AIDS patients has not been established at present. The suggested dose of both azoles is 400 mg/d and this should be continued for 6–8 weeks.

The decision to discontinue treatment should be based on clinical examination and the results of mycological and antigen tests. Lumbar punctures should be performed at 1-week intervals for the first 6 weeks of treatment. The return of CSF white cell counts, and protein and glucose levels to normal is helpful, but less reliable.

In addition to physical examination, blood and CSF specimens should be cultured and tested for antigen 1, 2, 3 and 6 months after treatment has ceased and thereafter at 12-month intervals.

AIDS PATIENTS

About 50% of AIDS patients with cryptococcosis will relapse within 6 months of successful completion of their initial treatment; a still greater proportion will relapse within 12 months. For this reason, long-term maintenance treatment is recommended for all patients with previous cryptococcosis.

At present, the combination of amphotericin and flucytosine is the preferred initial treatment for AIDS patients with meningeal or disseminated infection. The recommended dose of amphotericin is 0.5–1.0 mg/kg per day. The dose range for flucytosine is 75–150 mg/kg per day given as four divided doses and adjusted so as to maintain serum concentrations within the range 25–50 mg/l. This initial regimen should be given for at least 2 weeks. Thereafter, fluconazole (400 mg/d) or itraconazole (400 mg/d) may be substituted if the patient is much improved and may be capable of discharge from hospital. In milder cases, either fluconazole or itraconazole is acceptable as initial treatment.

Patients with high CSF antigen levels and continuing clinical signs of infection who cannot tolerate conventional amphotericin should be treated with liposomal amphotericin (AmBisome) (3.0 mg/kg per day) or fluconazole (400 mg/d). Amphotericin (with or without flucytosine) must be given to patients receiving azoles in whom recrudescent infection develops.

The optimum length of induction treatment and the total dose of amphotericin administered remains to be established. Most AIDS patients will require a total of at least 1.0–1.5 g of amphotericin as induction treatment. There are concerns about the myelotoxic effects of flucytosine. However, the relationship between drug dose, serum concentrations and toxic side effects is not clearly established.

More than 50% of AIDS patients with cryptococcosis relapse within 12 months of completing their initial treatment. This potential for relapse necessitates long-term use of antifungal drugs. Fluconazole (200–400 mg/d) is well tolerated and can be recommended. Itraconazole (200–400 mg/d) has also been used as long-term maintenance treatment, although late relapses have occurred following discontinuation of this drug.

Patients who have undergone successful treatment often relapse because of persistence of *C. neoformans* in the prostate. This site is asymptomatic, but it appears to account for relapses of infection in patients receiving less than 200 mg/d fluconazole, and indicates the need for higher dosing regimens.

12.7.3
Cutaneous
cryptococcosis

All patients with cutaneous cryptococcosis should be investigated for signs of disseminated infection. Lumbar puncture should be performed and radiographs of the underlying bone obtained. Blood should be tested for antigen. However, if the cutaneous lesion is the only manifestation of infection, the antigen test may well be negative.

If there is only one cutaneous lesion, surgical removal may be sufficient. However, it is advisable to give antifungal treatment with amphotericin or an azole.

13   Mucormycosis

13.1   Definition
The term mucormycosis (zygomycosis) is used to refer to infections due to moulds belonging to the Order Mucorales. These organisms can cause rhinocerebral, lung, gastrointestinal, cutaneous or disseminated infection in predisposed individuals, the different clinical forms often being associated with particular underlying conditions.

13.2   Geographical distribution
These infections are worldwide in distribution.

13.3   The causal organisms and their habitat
Many different organisms have been implicated, but the most common cause of human infection is *Rhizopus arrhizus* (*R. oryzae*). Other less frequent aetiological agents include *Absidia corymbifera*, *Cunninghamella bertholletiae*, *Rhizomucor pusillus* and *Saksenaea vasiformis*. These moulds are ubiquitous, thermotolerant and can be isolated in large numbers from soil or decomposing organic matter, such as fruit and bread. Their spores can often be found in the outside air.

Most infections follow inhalation of spores that have been released into the air, and the lungs and nasal sinuses are common initial sites of infection. Less often, infection follows ingestion or traumatic inoculation of organisms into the skin.

Nosocomial outbreaks of mucormycosis are not as common as hospital-related aspergillus infections, but have been reported in leukaemic patients. Nosocomial cutaneous infections with *R. rhizopodiformis* have been traced to contaminated dressings.

The major risk factors predisposing individuals to mucormycosis include uncontrolled diabetes mellitus, other forms of metabolic acidosis, burns and malignant haematological disorders. Treatment is seldom of benefit unless these underlying conditions can be corrected.

13.4   Clinical manifestations
Mucormycosis is an opportunistic infection and is seldom seen in normal persons. Various forms are recognized, each

of which is associated with particular underlying conditions. Like the aetiological agents of aspergillosis, the causal organisms of mucormycosis have a predilection for vascular invasion causing thrombosis, infarction and necrosis of tissue. The clinical hallmark of mucormycosis is the rapid onset of necrosis and fever. In most cases, progress is rapid and death follows unless treatment is initiated.

13.4.1 Rhinocerebral mucormycosis

The terms rhinocerebral and craniofacial mucormycosis are used to describe an infection that begins in the paranasal sinuses and then spreads to involve the orbit, face, palate or brain. This condition is most commonly seen in acidotic individuals, particularly those with uncontrolled diabetes mellitus, but it also occurs in leukaemic patients and organ transplant recipients. It is the most common clinical form of mucormycosis and often fatal within a week of onset if left untreated.

The initial symptoms include unilateral headache, nasal or sinus congestion or pain, and serosanguinous nasal discharge. Fever is also common. Most patients are not seen during the initial stage of local nasal and sinus infection. Two-thirds or more are lethargic or comatose by the time of their first examination.

If the infection has spread into the orbit, periorbital or perinasal swelling will progress to induration and discoloration. Ptosis, proptosis, dilatation and fixation of the pupil, and loss of vision may occur. Drainage of black pus from the eye is a useful diagnostic sign. From the orbit infection may spread into the brain leading to frontal lobe necrosis and abscess formation.

If the infection spreads into the palate, a black necrotic lesion is often found. This is an important diagnostic sign. Necrotic lesions may also be found on the nasal mucosa. Nasal septum or palatal perforation is frequent.

The CSF findings are nonspecific. The protein concentration may be slightly raised, but the glucose concentration is usually normal. There may be a modest mononuclear pleocytosis. CSF cultures are sterile.

The radiological findings are nonspecific, but are useful in delineating the extent of the infection. Diffuse craniofacial bone destruction is typical. CT and MR scans are helpful in defining the extent of bone and soft-tissue destruction, but are more useful in planning surgical intervention than in establishing a diagnosis. CT scans of the head often reveal sinus opacification, but other changes are minimal, even when there is massive orbital infection. MR scanning may be preferred for the diabetic patient for whom CT contrast agents may be contraindicated.

**13.4.2
Pulmonary
mucormycosis**

This condition is seldom diagnosed during life. Mucormycosis may develop in the lungs as a result of aspiration of infectious material, or following inhalation, or from haematogenous or lymphatic spread during dissemination. Most cases occur in leukaemic patients undergoing remission induction treatment. If untreated, haematogenous dissemination to other organs, particularly the brain, will often occur. The infection is fatal within 2–3 weeks.

The most common presentation is unremitting fever and the development or progression of lung infiltrates despite broad-spectrum antibacterial treatment. Haemoptysis and pleuritic chest pain are uncommon, but when present are helpful in suggesting a fungal infection. However, there are no characteristic symptoms or signs to distinguish mucormycosis from aspergillosis.

The chest radiographic findings are nonspecific, but the most common finding is focal or diffuse infiltrates that progress to consolidation, or cavitation, or wedge-shaped peripheral lesions, representing haemorrhagic infarction. Pleural effusion is uncommon.

**13.4.3
Gastrointestinal
mucormycosis**

This is an uncommon condition that has usually been encountered in malnourished infants or children. Lesions are most common in the stomach, colon and ileum. It is seldom diagnosed during life.

The symptoms are varied and depend on the site affected. Nonspecific abdominal pain and haematemesis are typical. Necrotic ulcers develop and peritonitis follows if intestinal perforation occurs. Intestinal mucormycosis is a fulminant illness ending in death within several weeks due to bowel infarction, sepsis, or haemorrhagic shock.

**13.4.4
Cutaneous
mucormycosis**

This is a particular problem in patients with burns in whom spread to underlying tissue is common. The initial signs include fever, swelling and changes in the appearance of the burn wound. The development of severe underlying necrosis and infarction in a burn should suggest the diagnosis.

Mucormycotic gangrenous cellulitis can follow other forms of trauma to the skin. In diabetic or immunosuppressed patients, cutaneous lesions may arise at an insulin injection site or a catheter insertion site. More massive trauma has been present in other patients, such as open fractures or crush injuries.

Necrotizing cutaneous mucormycosis has occurred in patients who have had contaminated surgical dressings applied to their skin.

Cutaneous lesions resembling ecthyma gangrenosum may develop following haematogenous dissemination of the fungus in immunosuppressed patients. The lesions begin as an erythematous, indurated painful cellulitis, then evolve into ulcers covered with a black eschar.

13.4.5 Disseminated mucormycosis

This may follow any of the four forms of mucormycosis described so far, but it is usually seen in neutropenic patients with pulmonary infection. Less commonly, dissemination occurs from the gastrointestinal tract, burns or other cutaneous lesions. The most common site of spread is the brain, but metastatic necrotic lesions have also been found in the spleen, heart and other organs. Disseminated mucormycosis is usually diagnosed after the patient has died of the infection. In occasional patients, metastatic cutaneous lesions permit an earlier diagnosis.

Cerebral infection following haematogenous dissemination is distinct from the rhinocerebral form of mucormycosis. It results in abscess formation and infarction. Patients present with sudden onset of focal neurological deficits or coma. Investigation of the CSF is unhelpful: protein, glucose and cell abnormalities are nonspecific and cultures are sterile. CT and MR scans are useful in locating the lesions.

13.4.6 Other forms of mucormycosis

Isolated mucormycotic brain lesions have been reported in a number of individuals, particularly parenteral drug abusers. The infection presents as a rapid deterioration in neurological status.

Other unusual focal forms of mucormycosis include endocarditis, osteomyelitis and pyelonephritis.

13.5

Differential diagnosis

Rhinocerebral mucormycosis is a dramatic and distinctive condition, but it can be confused with cavernous sinus thrombosis, bacterial orbital cellulitis or rhinocerebral aspergillosis or pseudallescheriosis.

The clinical manifestations of pulmonary mucormycosis cannot be distinguished from Gram-negative bacterial pneumonia, or aspergillosis or pseudallescheriosis.

13.6 **Essential investigations and their interpretation**

Because mucormycosis is such an aggressive infection, an early diagnosis is essential for successful treatment. It is, however, often difficult to obtain.

13.6.1
Microscopy

The microscopic demonstration of Mucorales in clinical material taken from necrotic lesions is more significant than their isolation in culture. These organisms can be distinguished from other moulds, such as *Aspergillus*, due to their characteristic broad, non-septate filaments with right-angled branching.

13.6.2
Culture

Nasal, palatal and sputum cultures are seldom helpful, but specimens should be sent for culture if the clinician suspects mucormycosis. Because the Mucorales are common contaminants, isolation of these organisms from sputum, or aspirated material from sinuses, or bronchial washings must be interpreted with caution. However, if the patient is diabetic or immunosuppressed, the isolation should not be ignored.

13.6.3
Serological tests

There are no routine serological tests for mucormycosis available at present.

13.7 **Management**

If treatment of mucormycosis is to be successful, underlying conditions must be controlled, infected necrotic tissue must be removed, and effective antifungal treatment must be administered. If surgical removal of infected tissue is not possible, the prognosis is poor.

Management of infection in the diabetic patient should consist of prompt correction of acidosis, rapid surgical debridement of infected and necrotic tissue, and administration of amphotericin. The drug is used at a dosage of at least 1.0 mg/kg per day and should be continued for 8–10 weeks.

In neutropenic patients with mucormycosis, amphotericin should be given at a dosage of 1.0 mg/kg per day from the outset as there is no time for gradual escalation (see Chapter 3). Immunosuppressive drugs should be reduced in dose or discontinued if this will not harm the patient.

Liposomal amphotericin (AmBisome) is much better tolerated than conventional amphotericin and doses as high as 3–5 mg/kg per day have been administered without significant side effects. Administration of the drug in this form has proved successful in some patients with rhinocerebral or other forms of mucormycosis.

In normal individuals, cutaneous mucormycosis has sometimes responded to surgical debridement alone, but amphotericin is advised.

Other antifungal drugs have no role in the management of mucormycosis.

With prompt diagnosis and treatment, 50% of diabetic patients with rhinocerebral mucormycosis can be cured. In contrast, few leukaemic patients with this infection recover.

14   Blastomycosis

14.1   Definition

The term blastomycosis is used to refer to infections due to the dimorphic fungus *Blastomyces dermatitidis*. Following inhalation this organism can cause chest infection in normal individuals, but it often spreads to involve other organs, in particular the skin and bones.

14.2   Geographical distribution

Most cases of blastomycosis have been reported from the South Central and South Eastern regions of North America, but the disease also occurs in Central and South America and parts of Africa.

14.3   The causal organism and its habitat

B. dermatitidis is a dimorphic fungus. It exists in nature as mycelium and as large, round budding cells in infected tissue.

It appears that the natural habitat of *B. dermatitidis* is the soil, although attempts to recover it have often proved unsuccessful. The fungus appears to survive best in wet soil of acid pH with a high organic content.

Unlike histoplasmosis and coccidioidomycosis, there is no accepted means of identifying subclinical and resolved infection in the human population, and this has also hindered attempts to delineate the endemic regions. Apart from epidemics, blastomycosis is much more common in men than women or children. It often occurs in individuals with an outdoor occupation or recreational interest.

14.4   Clinical manifestations

Infection follows inhalation of *B. dermatitidis* spores that have been released into the air. The lungs are the usual initial site of infection. In some cases the infection will resolve without dissemination to other organs, but in others it spreads to involve the skin, bone, prostate or other organs.

14.4.1 Pulmonary blastomycosis

Up to 50% of individuals develop no symptoms following inhalation of *B. dermatitidis* spores and their lung lesion is not detected until the infection has spread to other organs.

The remainder develop symptoms after an incubation period of 3–15 weeks.

In most cases blastomycosis is indolent in onset and patients present with chronic symptoms, such as cough, fever, malaise and weight loss, that have persisted for weeks or even months. Spontaneous resolution of the infection is uncommon. The lesions become more extensive, with continued suppuration and eventual necrosis and cavitation. Involvement of other sites is common in patients with chronic blastomycosis of the lungs.

Occasional patients present with an abrupt onset of infection, with the development of high fever, chills, productive cough, myalgia, arthralgia, and pleuritic chest pain. Often these patients appear to recover after 2–12 weeks of symptoms, but some will return months later with infection of other sites. Other patients with acute onset will fail to recover and will develop a chronic chest infection or disseminated infection.

Even a patient with hitherto indolent infection can develop a widespread interstitial infection that is fatal within 2 weeks of onset despite intensive treatment.

The chest radiographic findings are variable and not diagnostic. Lesions range from round, mass-like infiltrates with indistinct borders, to multiple nodular or segmental shadows involving most of the lung. Although pleuritic chest pain is not common, pleural involvement on radiographs is often seen, including thick irregular pleural-based lesions. Pleural effusions and cavitation of infiltrates are uncommon.

14.4.2
Cutaneous
blastomycosis

Haematogenous spread gives rise to cutaneous lesions in over 70% of patients with disseminated blastomycosis. These tend to be painless and present either as raised verrucous lesions with irregular borders, or as ulcers. The face, upper limbs, neck and scalp are the most frequent sites of involvement. Cutaneous lesions sometimes develop from lesions in underlying bone.

14.4.3
Osteoarticular
blastomycosis

Osteomyelitis occurs in about 30% of patients with disseminated blastomycosis. The spine, pelvis, cranial bones, ribs and long bones are the most common sites of infection. Patients often remain asymptomatic until the infection spreads into contiguous joints, or into adjacent soft tissue causing subcutaneous abscess formation. Infection of the spine can involve adjacent vertebral bodies with destruction of the intervening disc space.

The radiological findings are not specific and the well-defined osteolytic or osteoblastic lesions cannot be distinguished from those of other fungal or bacterial infections. Periosteal proliferation is unusual.

Arthritis occurs in up to 10% of patients with blastomycosis either as a result of haematogenous dissemination from the lung, or spread from a contiguous bone lesion. The symptoms include swelling, pain and limited movement in the affected joint.

**14.4.4
Genitourinary
blastomycosis**

The prostate, epididymis or testis are involved in 15–35% of men with disseminated blastomycosis. Patients with prostatic infection often present with obstruction or dysuria. Epididymitis presents as scrotal swelling with or without a draining sinus. Infection often spreads to the adjacent testis.

Venereal transmission of *B. dermatitidis* infection has resulted in self-limited genital ulceration or endometrial infection in the woman.

**14.4.5
Other forms of
disseminated
blastomycosis**

Haematogenous spread of infection to the brain has been reported in up to 10% of patients with disseminated blastomycosis. Manifestations of CNS infection include meningitis and spinal or brain abscess formation. Meningitis is indolent in onset and tends to occur late in the course of *B. dermatitidis* infection. It is often lethal and is indistinguishable from other forms of chronic meningitis such as tuberculosis or cryptococcosis.

Other organs, such as the adrenal glands or liver, are sometimes involved. Choroiditis and endophthalmitis have been reported.

14.5

Blastomycosis in special hosts

Although blastomycosis has been reported in patients with impaired T-cell-mediated immunological function, it is much less common than histoplasmosis or coccidioidomycosis. AIDS patients have developed fulminant blastomycosis with widespread dissemination following endogenous reactivation of previous infection.

14.6

Differential diagnosis

Tuberculosis of the skin, bone or genital tract, coccidioidomycosis of the lung, bone or meninges, and mucocutaneous paracoccidioidomycosis are other infections that can be confused with blastomycosis. However, the endemic regions for blastomycosis have almost no overlap with those of the other two fungal infections.

14.7 Essential investigations and their interpretation

14.7.1 Microscopy

Microscopic examination of wet preparations of pus, sputum, bronchial washings, urine or other clinical material can permit the diagnosis of blastomycosis if the characteristic large round cells with thick refractile walls and broad-based single buds are seen. Atypical *B. dermatitidis* cells can, however, be confused with other pathogens, such as single or non-budding cells of *Paracoccidioides brasiliensis*, *Histoplasma capsulatum* var. *duboisii*, and non-encapsulated cells of *Cryptococcus neoformans*.

14.7.2 Culture

The definitive diagnosis of blastomycosis depends on isolation of the fungus in culture. Identifiable mycelial colonies can be obtained after incubation at 25–30°C for 1–3 weeks, but cultures should be retained for 4 weeks before being discarded. The small globose single-celled spores are borne on simple lateral conidiophores. Subculture of the mycelial isolate on brain–heart–infusion agar or blood–glucose–cysteine agar at 37°C should result in the production of the unicellular form, confirming the identification. If a more rapid identification (24 h) is desired, the initial mycelial culture can be subjected to an exoantigen test.

14.7.3 Serological tests

Serological methods are of limited usefulness in the diagnosis of blastomycosis because of the high incidence of false-positive and false-negative reactions. The complement fixation test with unpurified antigen has been the least sensitive and least specific method. The immunodiffusion (ID) test is more specific, but negative reactions have been obtained in 10% of patients with disseminated infection and over 60% with localized infection. However, a positive reaction in the ID test can be considered diagnostic for blastomycosis.

14.8 Management

Amphotericin remains the drug of choice for patients with acute life-threatening infection and those with meningitis. The usual regimen is 0.4–0.5 mg/kg per day for 10 weeks. Patients with lung cavities or lesions in sites other than the lungs or skin may require more prolonged treatment. It is recommended that a total dose of 2 g should be given.

Oral itraconazole is the drug of choice for patients with indolent forms of blastomycosis. It should be given at a dosage of 200 mg/d with food for at least 3 months, and often as long as 6 months. If there is no obvious improvement, or if there are signs of progression, the dose should be increased to 400 mg/d given as two divided doses. Patients with serious infection who respond to initial treatment with amphotericin, can be changed to itraconazole for the remainder of their treatment. Oral ketoconazole (400 mg/d for 6 months) is almost as effective, but less well tolerated than itraconazole. Fluconazole (200–400 mg/d) appears to be less effective than itraconazole or ketoconazole.

Coccidioidomycosis

Definition
The term coccidioidomycosis is used to refer to infections
due to the dimorphic fungus *Coccidioides immitis*. Following
inhalation, this organism tends to cause a benign and transient chest infection in normal individuals, but it can proceed
to cause progressive infection of the lungs or more generalized infection.

Geographical distribution
Most cases of coccidioidomycosis have been reported from
the South Western USA, and parts of Central and South
America. However, the infection has also been diagnosed
outside these regions among individuals who had earlier
resided in or visited an endemic region.

The causal organism and its habitat
C. immitis is a dimorphic fungus. It exists in nature as a
mycelium which fragments into arthrospores. In tissue it
forms characteristic large, round, thick-walled spherules
which contain large numbers of endospores. Mycelium is
seldom produced in tissue, but is sometimes found in chronic
lung lesions.

C. immitis is a soil-inhabiting fungus with a restricted
geographical distribution. It is confined to certain hot, arid
parts of the South Western USA, and parts of Central and
South America. Climatic conditions in these regions consist
of a season of rainfall which favours mycelial proliferation in
the soil, and a long hot summer period during which large
numbers of arthrospores are produced and dispersed in dust
in the air. Dust storms can spread the organism far outside
its endemic regions. In parts of the endemic regions more
than 90% of inhabitants have had the infection.

Infection occurs when soil dust contaminated with arthrospores is inhaled. The lungs are the usual initial site of
infection.

Clinical manifestations
In most individuals inhalation of *C. immitis* arthrospores leads
to a benign and transient chest infection. In immunosup-

pressed or other predisposed individuals the infection can spread from the lungs to other sites and be fatal if left untreated.

**15.4.1
Primary
pulmonary
coccidioido-
mycosis**

About 60% of newly infected persons develop no symptoms following inhalation of *C. immitis* arthrospores. The remainder develop symptoms after an incubation period of 1–4 weeks. Most symptomatic patients develop a mild or moderate flu-like illness that resolves without treatment.

The most common symptoms are fever and pleuritic chest pain. Other symptoms include cough, malaise, headache, myalgia, night sweats and loss of appetite. Peripheral blood eosinophilia is often present.

Up to 50% of patients develop a mild, diffuse erythematous or maculopapular rash, covering the trunk and limbs, within the first few days of the onset of symptoms. More dramatic and persistent is the rash of erythema nodosum or erythema multiforme which occur in up to 30% of infected persons, but are more common in women. These signs occur up to 3 weeks after symptoms first appear and resolve over several weeks. Both are often accompanied by arthralgia in one or more joints.

The most common chest radiographic finding is segmental pneumonia seen in about 50% of cases. About 30% of infected individuals show minimal infiltrates, but 20% develop enlarged hilar lymph nodes or a pleural effusion. In addition, single or multiple nodules, as well as thick- or thin-walled cavities and enlarged mediastinal lymph nodes, can occur. In most cases, the radiographic abnormalities will resolve in 1–3 weeks.

**15.4.2
Chronic
pulmonary
coccidioido-
mycosis**

About 5% of infected individuals are left with residual signs of pulmonary coccidioidomycosis. In some cases, solid nodules are formed in the infiltrate. These are benign. In others, persistent thin-walled cavities develop. These often disappear within 2 years. Most patients are asymptomatic, but haemoptysis occurs in 25% of cases. Onset of fever, chest pain and dyspnoea is a sign that residual lung cavities have enlarged and ruptured into the pleural space causing a bronchopleural fistula or empyema.

In immunosuppressed patients with coccidioidomycosis, symptoms often persist and the patient can remain ill for months with fever, cough, chest pain and prostration. This acute progressive pneumonia can be fatal, often without disseminated infection.

Chronic progressive pneumonia can occur in patients who are not debilitated or immunosuppressed. This illness mimics tuberculosis. The symptoms include fever, cough, chest pain and weight loss. These patients have apical fibronodular lesions with small cavities.

15.4.3 Disseminated coccidioidomycosis

Fewer than 1% of infected individuals develop disseminated coccidioidomycosis. This is a progressive, often fatal illness that tends to occur in immunosuppressed or other predisposed groups of individuals. Men are five times more susceptible to dissemination than women, but the ratio is reversed if the woman is pregnant.

Dissemination tends to occur within a few weeks of the initial infection, although reactivation of a previous quiescent infection can occur if a patient should later become immunosuppressed. Most instances of disseminated coccidioidomycosis in AIDS patients have been due to reactivation.

The clinical manifestations of disseminated coccidioidomycosis range from a fulminant illness that is fatal within a few weeks if left untreated, to an indolent chronic illness that persists for months or years. One or more sites may be involved, but cutaneous, soft tissue, bone, joint and meningeal involvement is most common.

In immunosuppressed individuals, widespread rapid dissemination often occurs. Patients present with dramatic sweats, dyspnoea at rest, fever and weight loss. In most cases, chest radiographs reveal diffuse, miliary lesions. Patients undergo rapid clinical deterioration and die if left untreated.

Cutaneous and subcutaneous lesions are among the most common manifestations of disseminated coccidioidomycosis. Cutaneous lesions may be single or multiple and can persist for long periods. Their appearance is varied: verrucous papules, ulcers, erythematous plaques and nodules have been described. Underlying bone or joint lesions may be found.

Although most cutaneous lesions are due to haematogenous dissemination of the fungus, such lesions can follow direct inoculation. These often present as an indurated nodule with central ulceration. Lymphangitis may develop.

Osteomyelitis occurs in about 40% of patients with disseminated coccidioidomycosis. The spine, ribs, cranial bones, and ends of the long bones are the most common sites of infection. Patients often remain asymptomatic, but persistent dull pain may occur. Irregular lytic or sclerotic lesions are seen on radiographs. CT scans are useful in detecting asymptomatic lesions and should be performed in all patients with serious or disseminated infection. The infection may spread into contiguous joints causing arthritis, or into adjacent soft tissue, causing subcutaneous abscess formation. Draining sinuses often appear.

Meningitis is the most dreaded complication of coccidioidomycosis. It can occur without involvement of other sites or as part of a widespread disseminated infection. It often gives rise to hydrocephalus and is fatal if left untreated. The symptoms are nonspecific and insidious in onset. Persistent headache is often the earliest symptom. Mental changes, such as drowsiness and confusion, also occur. Other symptoms include loss of appetite, nausea and weight loss. Fever is minimal or absent in indolent cases.

Most patients with symptomatic meningitis have abnormal CSF findings, including raised protein concentration, lowered glucose concentration and a lymphocytic pleocytosis.

CT scans of the head are abnormal in most patients with meningeal coccidioidomycosis. The most common finding is ventricular enlargement. Hydrocephalus can be detected and monitored.

Other sites of infection include lymph nodes, liver, spleen and adrenal gland. Chorioretinitis, peritonitis, prostatitis and epididymitis are among the other unusual manifestations that have been reported.

15.5 Coccidioidomycosis in special hosts

15.5.1
AIDS patients

Coccidioidomycosis has become a serious problem in AIDS patients who have resided in, or travelled through, endemic regions. Most cases are found in AIDS patients still living in endemic regions, but cases have also occurred in AIDS patients who have not been in endemic regions for several years. AIDS patients may present with either localized coccidioidomycosis of the lungs or other organs, or widespread disseminated infection. The latter group often present with diffuse lung infiltrates and numerous other sites of infection. Few have survived for longer than a few months.

15.6 Differential diagnosis

The clinical presentation of primary pulmonary coccidioidomycosis is similar to that of blastomycosis and histoplasmosis, and also chlamydia and mycoplasma infection.

The radiological presentation in patients with residual

lung cavities due to *C. immitis* infection is similar to that of a number of other infectious and non-infectious conditions, including cryptococcosis, tuberculosis and bacterial lung abscess. In most of these other conditions the cavities have a thicker wall, or more extensive surrounding infiltrate.

The symptoms and clinical signs of chronic meningeal coccidioidomycosis are similar to those of cryptococcosis.

The large, cold abscesses that develop in soft tissue adjacent to *C. immitis* bone lesions can be mistaken for tuberculosis.

The diffuse lung infiltrates found in AIDS patients with coccidioidomycosis can be confused with *Pneumocystis carinii* infection.

15.7 Essential investigations and their interpretation

It is essential to inform the laboratory if a diagnosis of coccidioidomycosis is suspected, to ensure that proper precautions in handling of specimens and cultures are observed.

15.7.1 Microscopy

Microscopic examination of wet preparations of clinical material, such as sputum, pleural effusion fluid, pus or sediment of centrifuged CSF specimens, can permit the diagnosis of coccidioidomycosis if the characteristic large, thick-walled endospore-containing spherules are seen. Immature spherules and liberated endospores can, however, be confused with other pathogens, such as non-budding cells of *Blastomyces dermatitidis* or *Cryptococcus neoformans*.

15.7.2 Culture

The organism can be isolated from sputum, pleural effusion fluid, CSF sediment, pus and other specimens. Cultures must be set up in secure containers (tubes rather than plates) and handled with great care because of the danger of infection from the large concentrations of easily dispersed and highly infectious arthrospores. Identifiable mycelial colonies can be obtained after incubation at 25–30°C for 2–7 days, but cultures should be retained for at least 3 weeks before being discarded.

In culture, *C. immitis* must be distinguished from other moulds that produce arthrospores. The exoantigen test permits rapid identification. It is also useful for identifying atypical *C. immitis* isolates that fail to form arthrospores.

15.7.3 Skin tests

A positive coccidioidin or spherulin skin test result does not distinguish present from past infection. Conversion from a negative to a positive result is a sign of recent infection, because it occurs within 4 weeks of the onset of symptoms in 90–95% of patients. A negative result in an immunosuppressed patient does not rule out the diagnosis of coccidioidomycosis.

15.7.4
Serological tests

Serological tests are helpful in the diagnosis of coccidioidomycosis, although occasional cross-reactions occur in patients with histoplasmosis or blastomycosis.

Tests for the detection of immunoglobulin M (IgM) antibodies against *C. immitis* are most useful for diagnosing acute infection. These antibodies can be detected in most patients within 4 weeks of the onset of infection, but disappear within 2–6 months, even if the patient develops a disseminated infection. Immunoglobulin G (IgG) antibodies are most useful for detecting the later stages of coccidioidomycosis. These antibodies do not appear until 4–12 weeks after infection. In disseminated infection, IgG antibodies persist until death or until the patient recovers. The IgM titre is not significant, but IgG titres rise with progression of the infection and decline as the patient improves.

IgM antibodies can be detected with the latex particle agglutination (LPA) test, tube precipitin (TP) test, or immunodiffusion (ID) test. The LPA test is more sensitive, faster and simpler than the classical TP test, but gives at least 10% of false-positive reactions with serum and CSF specimens. For this reason a positive LPA test result must be confirmed with other methods.

The ID test with heated coccidioidin as antigen has replaced the TP test as the method of choice for diagnosing acute infection. It is more sensitive, faster and simpler than the TP method. Although uncommon, a positive ID reaction with CSF is an indication of meningitis.

IgG antibodies can be detected with the classical complement fixation (CF) test or using ID tests with filtered coccidioidin as antigen. In general, a rising CF titre (> 1 : 16) is consistent with spread of infection from the lungs. More than 50% of patients with disseminated infection have titres of more than 1 : 16. CF titres of 1 : 4 or 1 : 8 should not be considered as significant unless confirmed with a positive ID result.

The detection of antibodies in CSF is indicative of meningitis and remains the single most useful diagnostic test for that condition.

15.8 Management

**15.8.1
Primary
pulmonary
coccidioido-
mycosis**

Most immunocompetent persons have a benign, self-limited illness and will recover without antifungal treatment. However, infants, debilitated or immunosuppressed individuals, pregnant women and members of high-risk racial groups should be treated to prevent progression or dissemination of infection. Fewer than 5% of all infected patients require treatment.

Other factors that should determine the need for treatment of a primary infection in a noncompromised patient include: persistent symptoms lasting more than 6 weeks; prostration; widespread, enlarging or persistent lung involvement; persistent hilar or mediastinal lymph node enlargement; rising or elevated titres ($> 1 : 16$) of IgG antibodies.

If antifungal treatment is indicated in a patient with primary coccidioidomycosis, amphotericin should be used. The usual regimen is 0.4–0.6 mg/kg per day. Provided the patient has stabilized, 0.8–1.0 mg/kg can be given at 48-h intervals. It is recommended that treatment should be continued until a total dose of 0.5–1.5 g has been given.

**15.8.2
Chronic
pulmonary
coccidioido-
mycosis**

Patients with small, nonprogressive cavities should be observed until spontaneous resolution occurs. Those with large or progressive cavities often require surgical resection. This is indicated if the cavities are near the pleural surface, or if serious and persistent haemoptysis, or bacterial superinfection is a problem. It is also advisable to give a short 4-week course of amphotericin (0.4–0.6 mg/kg per day), commencing about 2 weeks before the surgical procedure, to prevent complications such as the development of a bronchopleural fistula or empyema.

Patients with chronic progressive apical infiltrates resembling tuberculosis present a difficult problem. Infection tends to be indolent and although amphotericin (0.4–0.6 mg/kg per day) often arrests progression, relapse is common after treatment is discontinued. Use of oral ketoconazole (400 mg/d) has led to clinical improvement in up to 25% of patients who have not received previous treatment. Higher doses of this drug are more toxic and no more effective than 400 mg/d. It should be continued, in patients who respond, for at least 6–12 months. Ketoconazole also appears useful in delaying relapse after amphotericin treatment.

**15.8.3
Disseminated
coccidioido-
mycosis**

The drug of choice for patients with disseminated coccidioidomycosis is amphotericin. The usual adult dose is
1.0–1.5 mg/kg per day. Treatment should be continued
until a total dose of 2.5–3.0 g has been given. The results of
treatment are often disappointing and relapse is a common
problem.

Oral ketoconazole (400 mg/d) has been used to treat disseminated coccidioidomycosis, but relapse rates of 25–30%,
even after 12 months of treatment, have been reported. The
best results have been reported in patients with cutaneous
lesions or joint effusions.

Itraconazole (400 mg/d) appears to be at least as effective
as ketoconazole and better tolerated. However, long periods
of treatment are often required. Fluconazole (400 mg/d)
also appears promising for patients with non-meningeal disseminated coccidioidomycosis. Treatment with these drugs
should be continued for at least 6–12 months after the
infection is considered inactive.

Surgical debridement is important in the management of
osteomyelitis and in the diagnosis and drainage of soft tissue
lesions.

Amphotericin is the most appropriate initial treatment for
AIDS patients with coccidioidomycosis. This initial regimen
should be continued until a total dose of 1.0 g has been
given. Thereafter, itraconazole (400 mg/d) or fluconazole
(400 mg/d) may be substituted if the patient has improved.

**15.8.4
Meningitis**

Amphotericin remains the treatment of choice for this condition. Total courses of between 1.0 and 4.0 g of parenteral
amphotericin are given, combined with intrathecal or intracisternal administration of the drug. Intracisternal injection is to be preferred to lumbar intrathecal injection because
of the risk of development of chronic lumbar arachnoiditis.
In some cases, an indwelling intraventricular reservoir has
been used, but this is liable to complications. If hydrocephalus is present, a ventriculoperitoneal shunt should
be inserted. However, it must be remembered that drugs
administered into the drained portion of the CSF will be lost
into the general circulation.

The dosage regimen and duration of local treatment
depend on the clinical course. For the first few weeks,
intracisternal or intrathecal injections should be given two or
three times per week, with the dose increased as tolerated to
0.5–1.0 mg. Doses as high as 1.0–1.5 mg at 48-h intervals
for the first 6 months have sometimes been advocated.

Provided the patient's condition has improved, the interval between injections can be increased. Treatment should not be discontinued until CF test results on lumbar CSF specimens are negative and CSF glucose concentrations have been normal for several months.

Both intracisternal and intraventricular amphotericin injections lead to headache, nausea and fever. Symptoms begin within 30 min after injection and last for several hours. Hydrocortisone sodium succinate (25 mg) should be added to the injection to reduce drug-related inflammation.

Oral ketoconazole has been used to treat meningeal coccidioidomycosis, but a dose of at least 1200 mg/d has been required and intolerance has been a frequent problem. It should not be used unless intrathecal treatment with amphotericin is impossible. Itraconazole (400 mg/d) and fluconazole (400 mg/d) have been used in small numbers of patients with some success. Long-term treatment is required.

Treatment of meningeal coccidioidomycosis is best regarded as suppressive rather than curative, and long-term follow up after treatment is required.

16   Histoplasmosis

16.1

Definition

The term histoplasmosis is used to refer to infections due to the dimorphic fungus *Histoplasma capsulatum*. Following inhalation, this organism tends to cause a mild and transient chest infection in normal individuals, but it can proceed to cause chronic infection of the lungs or more widespread infection in predisposed patients.

16.2

Geographical distribution

Although histoplasmosis has a global distribution, it is most prevalent in the central region of North America and in Central and South America. Other endemic regions include Africa, Australia and parts of East Asia, in particular India and Malaysia.

16.3

The causal organism and its habitat

H. capsulatum is a dimorphic fungus. It exists in nature as a mycelium. In tissue it forms small round budding cells.

Two varieties of *H. capsulatum* are recognized: var. *capsulatum* and var. *duboisii*. The two varieties are indistinguishable in their mycelial (saprophytic) forms, but differ in their parasitic forms. The cells of the tissue form of var. *duboisii* are much larger and have thicker walls than those of var. *capsulatum*.

The natural habitat of *H. capsulatum* is soil enriched with bird or bat droppings. If contaminated soil or bird roosts are disturbed during building construction or demolition, this can lead to enormous numbers of spores being dispersed in the air and result in large numbers of individuals being infected. Numerous epidemic outbreaks of histoplasmosis have been reported from the USA. Bat-roosting sites, such as caves, are also important sources of *H. capsulatum*, particularly in the tropics.

It is estimated that 500 000 persons are infected per annum in the USA, making it the most common endemic mycosis. In certain endemic parts of the USA, more than 80% of the population have had subclinical and resolved infection.

Although infections due to *H. capsulatum* var. *duboisii* have been confined to the central region of the African continent (and termed African histoplasmosis), infections with var. *capsulatum* have also been reported from parts of that continent.

16.4

Clinical manifestations

In most persons, inhalation of *H. capsulatum* spores leads to a transient chest infection which subsides without treatment. In some individuals, however, the organism can cause chronic lung infection or more widespread infection. This is a progressive, often fatal, illness.

16.4.1
Acute
pulmonary
histoplasmosis

Most normal individuals develop no symptoms following inhalation of low levels of *H. capsulatum* spores. Inhalation of higher levels of spores results in an acute symptomatic infection after an incubation period of 1–3 weeks.

The most common symptoms are fever, chills, headache, myalgia, loss of appetite, cough and retrosternal or pleuritic chest pain. About 10% of patients present with arthritis or severe arthralgia associated with erythema nodosum. These manifestations can persist for several months.

Chest radiographs reveal small, scattered, nodular infiltrates. Hilar lymph node enlargement is often evident and pleural effusion may be found. The infiltrates tend to heal over several months leaving scattered calcifications throughout both lung fields.

Most persons will recover without treatment, their symptoms disappearing within 1–3 weeks. Return to full strength can take several months.

Healing of a localized infiltrate may result in the development of a residual round nodule, often termed a histoplasmoma, that enlarges as fibrous material is deposited around the lesion. If calcification is absent, these benign lesions cannot be distinguished from a neoplasm on chest radiographs.

Individuals reinfected with *H. capsulatum* develop a similar illness, but this is milder and occurs after a much shorter incubation period (less than 1 week). These patients present with abrupt onset of malaise, headache, chills, fever and cough, but the symptoms are less severe and of shorter duration. The chest radiograph signs are different. Multiple, small, interstitial miliary nodules are present, but there is no mediastinal lymph node enlargement and pleural effusions are not seen. Late calcification does not occur. The illness tends to resolve without treatment.

Following inhalation of *H. capsulatum*, the organism gains access to the alveolar and interstitial lung tissue and then spreads through the lymphatics to the lymph nodes, causing hilar or mediastinal lymphadenitis that persists long after the infiltrates have resolved. Mediastinal fibrosis can develop and lead to tracheal, bronchial or vascular obstruction. Enlarged mediastinal nodes can erode into adjacent pericardium causing pericarditis.

16.4.2
Chronic
pulmonary
histoplasmosis

This slowly progressive illness usually occurs in middle-aged men with underlying chronic obstructive lung disease. It first manifests itself as transient, segmental interstitial infiltrates that heal without treatment, but may progress to chronic fibrosis and cavitation with destruction of significant amounts of lung tissue. If left untreated, death can result from progressive lung failure.

The initial symptoms often include cough or increased cough (often productive), fever, weight loss, malaise and pleuritic chest pain. Often the patient has been ill for weeks or months. The main radiological findings are interstitial infiltrates in the apical segments of the upper lobes of the lung.

Interstitial infiltrates often disappear, but cavitation can occur. If this is left untreated the course is one of insidious tissue destruction resulting in haemoptysis, recurrent bacterial infection with abscess formation, and death.

The most prominent symptoms in patients with cavitary histoplasmosis are cough and sputum production. Other symptoms include fever, chest pain, fatigue and weight loss. Haemoptysis develops in more than 30% of patients. The clinical findings can mimic tuberculosis.

Chest radiographs will reveal progressive infiltration and cavitation. Cavities with walls thicker than 3 mm in diameter are associated with established and continuing infection. Lesions are more common in the right upper lobe than in the left, but bilateral lesions develop in about 25% of patients and, in time, the infection will spread to the lower lobes. Pleural effusion is uncommon, but pleural thickening adjacent to lesions is found in 50% of patients.

16.4.3
Disseminated
histoplasmosis

This is a progressive, often lethal illness, that tends to develop in immunosuppressed patients or other predisposed groups of individuals, particularly infants and persons over 55 years of age.

The clinical manifestations of disseminated histoplasmosis

range from a fulminant illness that is fatal within a few weeks if left untreated (often seen in infants and immunosuppressed patients) to an indolent, chronic illness that can affect a wide range of sites and persist for months or years.

Infants and immunosuppressed patients often present with fever, chills, prostration, malaise, loss of appetite and weight loss. Symptoms lasting more than 3 weeks suggest disseminated infection because most cases of acute histoplasmosis resolve in less than 2 weeks.

The liver and spleen are enlarged and liver function tests are abnormal. Anaemia is common. Chest radiographs are often normal, but if abnormal, diffuse interstitial infiltrates are more common than focal infiltrates. Pleural effusions are uncommon. Mucosal lesions can occur, but are much less common than in patients with indolent progression of the illness.

In nonimmunosuppressed individuals, disseminated histoplasmosis follows an indolent, chronic course. Often chest radiographs are normal. Hepatic infection is common, but enlargement of the liver and spleen is not as pronounced as in patients with fulminant infection. Adrenal gland destruction is a common problem.

Mucosal ulcers are found in over 60% of patients with indolent infection. The mouth and throat are often affected, but lesions also occur on the lip, nose, glans penis and other sites. Most patients have a single lesion, painless at first, with a characteristic, distinct heaped-up margin.

Meningitis or focal cerebral lesions occur in 10–25% of patients with indolent disseminated histoplasmosis. The main symptoms are headache and mental changes. Often patients have had these symptoms for several months or longer before diagnosis. Most patients have abnormal CSF findings including elevated protein concentration, lowered glucose concentration and a mild pleocytosis. CT scans will reveal cerebral lesions.

Other manifestations of chronic disseminated histoplasmosis include endocarditis (often with large vegetations) and mucosal ulcerations in the gastrointestinal tract. The latter often present as bleeding, perforation, or less commonly, obstruction.

**16.4.4
African
histoplasmosis**

The clinical manifestations of *H. capsulatum* var. *duboisii* infection differ in a number of respects from those of var. *capsulatum* infection described in the preceding sections. The illness is indolent in onset and the predominant sites affected are the skin and bones. Those with more wide-spread infection involving the liver, spleen and other organs have a febrile wasting illness that is fatal within weeks or months if left untreated.

Bone lesions are often painless. The spine, ribs, cranial bones, sternum and long bones are the most common sites of infection. Multiple lesions are often found. The infection can spread into contiguous joints causing arthritis, or into adjacent soft tissue, causing a purulent subcutaneous abscess. Other cutaneous manifestations of African histoplasmosis are subcutaneous granulomata and nodular or papular lesions. Papules are common on the face and trunk. Both nodules and papules often enlarge and ulcerate.

16.5 Histoplasmosis in special hosts

16.5.1 AIDS patients

Disseminated histoplasmosis is a serious problem in AIDS patients who have resided in, or travelled through, endemic regions. Fever and weight loss are the most common presenting symptoms. Up to 25% of infected patients have an enlarged liver and spleen and a similar proportion have anaemia, leucopenia and thrombocytopenia. Mucosal lesions are uncommon.

Chest radiographs reveal diffuse interstitial or reticulonodular infiltrates in about 50% of AIDS patients with histoplasmosis. About 30% have normal radiographs on admission. Meningitis, although still uncommon, occurs more commonly than in other groups of patients. Although the illness is usually gradual in onset, up to 10% of patients have presented with disseminated intravascular coagulation, often with multiple organ failure leading to rapid death.

16.6 Differential diagnosis

The clinical presentation of acute pulmonary histoplasmosis is similar to that of many other conditions, including chlamydia, legionella and mycoplasma infection.

The clinical and radiological presentation of chronic pulmonary histoplasmosis is similar to that of tuberculosis and coccidioidomycosis.

16.7 Essential investigations and their interpretation

16.7.1 Microscopy

Microscopic examination of wet preparations of clinical material, such as sputum or pus, is not a suitable method for the diagnosis of histoplasmosis. All material should be examined as stained smears.

If microscopic examination of peripheral blood smears, or stained histopathological sections, or other specimens from individuals who have resided in, or visited, endemic regions reveal small oval budding cells (often clustered within mononuclear phagocytic cells), the diagnosis of histoplasmosis should be suspected. *H. capsulatum* var. *capsulatum* cells can, however, be confused with other pathogens, such as *Penicillium marneffei*, as well as with atypical small cells of *Blastomyces dermatitidis* and small, non-encapsulated cells of *Cryptococcus neoformans*.

If clinical specimens contain large, thick-walled cells and the patient has resided in or visited the African continent, *H. capsulatum* var. *duboisii* should be suspected as the pathogen.

Organisms tend to be much more abundant in peripheral blood smears and bronchial washings from AIDS patients.

16.7.2
Culture

The definitive diagnosis of histoplasmosis depends on isolation of the fungus in culture. Incubation of cultures should be at 25–30°C for 4–6 weeks. It is often difficult to distinguish the mycelial colonies of *H. capsulatum* from those of *B. dermatitidis* and species of *Chrysosporium* and *Sepedonium*. Unequivocal identification of a mycelial isolate as *H. capsulatum* requires conversion to the yeast form, which can take 3–6 weeks, or exoantigen testing which permits specific identification within 48–72 h.

H. capsulatum has been isolated from blood, sputum, bone marrow, pus, tissue and other specimens. Lysis centrifugation has been the most useful method for recovering it from blood. CSF cultures are positive in 25–50% of patients with meningitis.

16.7.3
Skin tests

The histoplasmin skin test is not recommended for diagnosis of histoplasmosis, because a positive result does not distinguish present from past infection. Nor does a negative result rule out active infection. Moreover, it can induce the formation of antibodies, making the results of subsequent serological tests difficult to interpret.

16.7.4
Serological tests

Serological tests are useful in the diagnosis of histoplasmosis. The immunodiffusion (ID) and complement fixation (CF) tests, with histoplasmin as antigen, are positive in about 80% of patients, including those with acute, self-limited infection. In disseminated histoplasmosis, serological tests are positive less often in immunosuppressed patients.

The CF test is more sensitive than ID in histoplasmosis. No more than 1% of patients with a negative CF test result will give a positive ID reaction. However, the CF test is not altogether specific and cross-reactions can occur in patients with blastomycosis or coccidioidomycosis. Nonspecific CF tests tend to give titres of 1:8–1:32. However, similar titres are often obtained in tests with serum from patients with proven histoplasmosis. CF titres of more than 1:32 or rising titres in serial specimens are considered a more convincing sign of active infection.

The ID test is more specific, but less sensitive than CF for histoplasmosis. Using histoplasmin as antigen, two major precipitin bands can be detected. The H band is specific for active histoplasmosis, but only occurs in 10–25% of patients. The M band can be detected in up to 85% of patients with active infection, but may also be found in patients with past infection, or in those who have had a recent histoplasmin skin test. Because the H and M bands are specific for histoplasmosis, the ID test provides a more specific diagnosis with serum specimens that have low CF titres or that cross-react in CF tests.

Antigen detection is a sensitive method for diagnosis of disseminated histoplasmosis in AIDS patients. Circulating *H. capsulatum* antigen can be detected in the blood and urine of 80–100% of these patients. Antigenuria has been detected in 25–50% of patients with less serious infection. Antigen levels fall in patients receiving antifungal treatment and rise in those who have relapsed. Antigen has also been detected in CSF specimens from patients with meningitis.

16.8 Management

16.8.1 Acute pulmonary histoplasmosis

Few patients presenting with this form of histoplasmosis require treatment. In most cases spontaneous improvement has begun before the condition is diagnosed.

Patients with progressive and gross enlargement of hilar or mediastinal lymph nodes should be treated to prevent atelectasis and mediastinal fibrosis. Neither corticosteroid administration nor antifungal treatment have been beneficial in patients with mediastinal fibrosis, and surgical intervention to relieve obstruction has often proved difficult.

The treatment of choice in the few patients who require

active management is amphotericin (for 2–4 weeks) and bed rest with an adequate diet.

16.8.2 Chronic pulmonary histoplasmosis

If patients are seen in the initial stages of this illness and there is no cavitation and symptoms are mild, antifungal treatment can be withheld, provided signs of healing are observed. If symptoms progress or persist, antifungal treatment must be given. Surgical resection is no longer recommended.

Oral itraconazole (400 mg/d for 6 months) appears to be the drug of choice for most patients with this condition. Oral ketoconazole (400 mg/d for 6–12 months) can be used, but it is less well tolerated. Patients whose compliance with prolonged treatment is poor, and those requiring H_2-antagonists or other drugs that impair itraconazole or ketoconazole absorption, should receive amphotericin. The usual regimen is 0.4–0.5 mg/kg per day for 10 weeks (0.8–1.0 mg/kg can be given at 48-h intervals). Patients should be followed up for at least 12 months after treatment is discontinued.

16.8.3 Disseminated histoplasmosis

All patients should receive antifungal treatment, even those with a single focal lesion.

Nonimmunosuppressed patients with indolent, nonmeningeal infection can be treated with oral itraconazole (400 mg/d) or ketoconazole (400 mg/d) for 6–12 months. Patients with fulminant or severe infection should be treated with amphotericin (0.5–0.6 mg/kg per day) for 10 weeks. Infants should receive 1.0 mg/kg for at least 6 weeks.

The management of AIDS patients with disseminated histoplasmosis presents special problems. Even if initial treatment is successful, these patients often relapse when amphotericin is discontinued. One approach is to administer a 1.0–2.0 g dose of amphotericin over 6–8 weeks and follow this with indefinite maintenance treatment: an infusion of 1.0 mg/kg of amphotericin at 1- or 2-week intervals has proved successful. However, the risk of long-term toxic side effects must be borne in mind.

Oral ketoconazole should not be used for the initial treatment of AIDS patients with histoplasmosis. Nor can it be recommended for long-term maintenance treatment. Oral itraconazole (200 mg/d) appears promising for long-term suppressive treatment.

17   Paracoccidioidomycosis

Definition

The term paracoccidioidomycosis is used to refer to infections due to the dimorphic fungus *Paracoccidioides brasiliensis*. Following inhalation this organism can cause chest infection in normal individuals, but it often spreads to other organs causing chronic ulcerated granulomatous lesions on the buccal, nasal and gastrointestinal mucosa. The lymph nodes are often involved and sometimes cutaneous lesions appear.

17.2

Geographical distribution

Most cases of paracoccidioidomycosis have been reported from South and Central America, although it has been diagnosed outside these regions in individuals who had earlier resided in or visited an endemic region.

17.3

The causal organism and its habitat

P. brasiliensis is a dimorphic fungus. It grows in nature as a mycelium, but in tissue it forms large oval or globose cells with characteristic multiple buds encircling the mother cell.

    P. brasiliensis has been recovered from occasional soil specimens, but understanding of its natural habitat remains limited. In South and Central America, paracoccidioidomycosis is most frequently encountered in regions classified as subtropical mountain forests.

    The highest incidence of clinical paracoccidioidomycosis occurs in men with outdoor occupations between the ages of 20 and 50 years.

17.4

Clinical manifestations

Inhalation of *P. brasiliensis* spores results in infection of the lungs. In some cases the condition will resolve without dissemination to other organs, but in others it spreads to involve the mucosa, skin or other organs. Two or more sites may be involved in a particular patient. The disease is often indolent in onset, appearing long after an individual has left an endemic region.

**17.4.1
Pulmonary
paracoccidioido-
mycosis**

In most cases paracoccidioidomycosis is indolent in onset and patients present with chronic symptoms, such as cough, fever, night sweats, malaise and weight loss.

The chest radiographic findings are characteristic, but not diagnostic. Multiple bilateral infiltrates are common. Fibrosis and cavitation occur in long-standing cases. Calcification, pleural effusion and hilar lymph node enlargement are uncommon. The infection must be distinguished from histoplasmosis and tuberculosis.

**17.4.2
Mucocutaneous
paracoccidioido-
mycosis**

This is the second most common clinical form of paracoccidioidomycosis. Indeed, the high incidence of oral lesions has led to suggestions that direct implantation of the organism into the mouth may occur.

The mouth and nose are the most usual mucosal sites of infection. Painful ulcerated lesions develop on the gums, tongue, lips or palate and can progress over weeks or months, interfering with eating. Perforation of the palate or nasal septum may occur. Laryngeal lesions can lead to scar formation and ulceration resulting in hoarseness and stridor.

Cutaneous lesions often appear on the face around the mouth and nose, although patients with severe infection can have widespread scattered lesions. Small papular or nodular lesions enlarge over weeks or months into plaques with an elevated, well-defined margin. Verrucous lesions or ulcers with a rolled border may develop.

**17.4.3
Lympho-
nodular
paracoccidioido-
mycosis**

Lymphadenitis is common in younger patients. Cervical and submandibular chains are the most obvious manifestation, but mediastinal and femoral nodes may be involved. Lymph nodes may progress to form cold abscesses with sinuses that drain onto the overlying skin.

**17.4.4
Disseminated
paracoccidioido-
mycosis**

Haematogenous spread of *P. brasiliensis* can result in widespread disseminated infection. Manifestations include nodular or ulcerated lesions of the small or large intestine, hepatic lesions, adrenal gland destruction, osteomyelitis, arthritis, endophthalmitis, and meningoencephalitis or focal cerebral lesions.

Symptoms of disseminated infection depend on the rate of progress and duration of disease. Fever is more common in acute cases. Profound weight loss and prostration often occur late in the course. Anaemia develops as the infection proceeds.

17.5

Differential diagnosis

Mucocutaneous leishmaniasis is endemic in the same regions as paracoccidioidomycosis and can cause similar lesions. The clinical and radiological manifestations of *P. brasiliensis* infection of the lungs can be confused with tuberculosis or histoplasmosis.

17.6

Essential investigations and their interpretation

17.6.1
Microscopy

Microscopic examination of wet preparations of pus, sputum, crusts from granulomatous lesions and other clinical material can permit the diagnosis of paracoccidioidomycosis if the characteristic large, round cells with multiple peripheral buds are seen. However, these are usually present as single cells or chains of cells and often cannot be differentiated from other fungal pathogens.

17.6.2
Culture

The definitive diagnosis of paracoccidioidomycosis depends on isolation of the fungus in culture. Mycelial colonies can be obtained after incubation at 25–30°C for 2–3 weeks, but cultures should be retained for 4 weeks before being discarded. Mycelial cultures seldom sporulate, but subculture of the isolate on blood agar at 37°C should result in production of the unicellular form. If more rapid identification is required (24 h), the initial mycelial culture can be subjected to an exoantigen test.

17.6.3
Serological tests

Serological tests are useful for the diagnosis of paracoccidioidomycosis. These tests have also been helpful for following the effect of treatment.

The complement fixation test is positive in more than 90% of patients with paracoccidioidomycosis, higher titres being obtained in those with more severe infection. However, cross-reactions can occur with serum from patients with blastomycosis, histoplasmosis, sporotrichosis and several other infections.

The immunodiffusion test is positive in 80–90% of patients with paracoccidioidomycosis. Although cross-reactions can occur in patients with histoplasmosis, these are uncommon.

Titres of antibodies decline on successful treatment,

precipitins being the first to disappear. However, low titres may persist for a long time after cure of the infection.

17.7 Management

All patients with paracoccidioidomycosis require antifungal treatment, because spontaneous resolution does not occur. Long-term follow-up is important in all cases because of the high incidence (25%) of late relapse.

Itraconazole is the drug of choice for the treatment of paracoccidioidomycosis. The usual regimen is 50–100 mg/d given for 6 months. Late relapse has been uncommon. Oral ketoconazole is almost as effective, but less well tolerated than itraconazole. The usual dose is 200–400 mg/d given for up to 12 months (or for a minimum of 6 months after all clinical signs of infection have disappeared). The role of fluconazole has not been established.

If absorption of itraconazole or ketoconazole is a problem, treatment with amphotericin and a sulphonamide (such as sulphadiazine) should be prescribed. Amphotericin (1.0 mg/kg per day) should be administered for the first 4–8 weeks. Thereafter, treatment with sulphadiazine should be continued for a further 6 months or longer. The usual adult dose of sulphadiazine is 500–1000 mg at 4–6-h intervals. Children should receive 60–100 mg/kg per day in divided doses.

If the cost of treatment is a significant consideration, sulphadiazine can be used as the sole treatment for paracoccidioidomycosis.

18   Chromoblastomycosis

18.1

Definition

The term chromoblastomycosis (chromomycosis) is used to refer to a chronic localized infection of the skin and subcutaneous tissue most often involving the limbs and characterized by raised, crusted lesions. It may be caused by a number of brown-pigmented (dematiaceous) fungi.

18.2

Geographical distribution

The disease is encountered mainly in arid parts of tropical and subtropical regions. Most cases occur in Central and South America, but chromoblastomycosis has also been reported in South Africa, Asia and Australia.

18.3

The causal organisms and their habitat

The disease is caused by various dematiaceous fungi, to which a number of names have been given. There is therefore a great deal of confusion in the nomenclature used by various authors.

The most frequently involved aetiological agents, in descending order, are *Phialophora verrucosa, Fonsecaea pedrosoi, Fonsecaea compacta, Cladosporium carrionii* and *Rhinocladiella aquaspersa (Ramichloridium cerophilum)*. Sporadic cases of chromoblastomycosis can also be caused by other dematiaceous moulds. These organisms form characteristic thick-walled dark brown muriform sclerotic cells in tissue.

The aetiological agents of chromoblastomycosis are widespread in the environment, being found in soil, wood and decomposing plant matter. Human infection usually follows the traumatic inoculation of the fungus into the skin. The disease is most prevalent in rural parts of warmer climates where individuals go barefoot. There is no human-to-human transmission.

Chromoblastomycosis is unusual in children and adolescents. Except in Japan, men contract the disease much more frequently than women, reflecting the importance of occupational exposure.

Infection usually follows the traumatic introduction of the

fungus into the skin. Minor trauma, such as cuts or wounds due to thorns or wood splinters, is often sufficient.

Clinical manifestations

18.4

The lesions are usually unilateral and occur mainly on the exposed parts of the body, particularly the feet and lower legs. Other less common sites include the hands, arms, shoulders and neck. The initial lesion is a painless papule or nodule on an erythematous and occasionally verrucous base. The condition may also present as an abscess surrounded by infiltration or as a psoriasiform lesion with erythema and scaling. As the disease develops, the affected limb becomes enlarged. Small satellite nodules may occur at the edge of the original lesion. Itching often occurs and it may be severe.

The primary lesion develops very slowly, its diameter increasing by only 1–2 mm per year. It is firm and elastic in consistency, coloured red or violet verging on grey. There is a warty, papillomatous margin surrounding a centre that may be flat, smooth or scaly and showing areas of scarring.

Later in the disease the lesion may become pedunculated or ulcerated (if bacterial superinfection occurs). However, the lesions usually retain a warty, dry character.

Secondary lesions may appear, especially along the lymphatics draining the site of infection; here again, development is slow and symptoms are few. The lymph nodes are only involved if there is superimposed bacterial infection.

In some cases the skin lesions may spread and involve an entire limb. In other cases there is spontaneous resolution, leaving behind scars that are atrophic and abnormally pigmented or, by contrast, hypertrophic and contracting scars.

Cutaneous dissemination is rare, but may follow auto-inoculation due to scratching. Lymphatic or haematogenous spread may also occur. In elderly patients the lesions may spread to involve the skin of the trunk whereas the scalp is rarely involved. The nails may also be damaged as a result of infection of the matrix and nail bed.

Rare complications of chromoblastomycosis include carcinomatous transformation. Metastatic lesions may occur in the oral mucosa, lymph nodes, bones and other tissues.

Usually lesions on the upper limbs are erythematosquamous, psoriasiform, and of low relief, whereas those on the lower limbs are more exuberant. The latter may be associated with sclerosing inflammation of the subcutaneous tissue and result in elephantiasis.

18.5

Differential diagnosis

In endemic areas the unilateral development of vegetative, atrophic and scarred lesions on a lower limb is suggestive of chromoblastomycosis.

The condition must be distinguished from a number of other fungal infections including blastomycosis, lobomycosis, paracoccidioidomycosis, phaeohyphomycosis, rhinosporidiosis and sporotrichosis. It must also be differentiated from prototohecosis, leishmaniasis, verrucous tuberculosis, certain leprous lesions and syphilis.

On the upper limbs the erythematosquamous lesions can be confused with psoriasis or subacute or discoid lupus erythematosus.

Mycological and histological investigations are indispensable for confirmation of the diagnosis.

18.6

Essential investigations and their interpretation

18.6.1
Microscopy

Microscopic examination of wet preparations of pus, scrapings or crusts from lesions can permit the diagnosis of chromoblastomycosis if clusters of the characteristic small, round, thick-walled, brown-pigmented sclerotic cells are seen. These cells are often divided by longitudinal and transverse septa.

18.6.2
Culture

The definitive diagnosis of chromoblastomycosis depends on the isolation of the aetiological agent in culture. Identifiable olive green–brownish black mycelial colonies can be obtained after incubation at 25–30°C for 1–2 weeks, but cultures should be retained for 4 weeks before being discarded. Identification of the individual aetiological agents is difficult.

18.7

Management

Chromoblastomycosis is a difficult condition to treat. Surgical excision should be reserved for small lesions. It carries a high risk of local dissemination and should only be attempted in conjunction with antifungal treatment.

There is no ideal antifungal treatment for chromoblastomycosis. The most commonly used drug is flucytosine (150–200 mg/kg per day given as four divided doses), but resistance is a frequent problem during long-term treatment.

Much better results have been obtained when flucytosine (4.0 g/d given as four divided doses) is combined with oral thiabendazole (1.0 g/d given as two divided doses). Treatment should be continued for at least 1 month after clinical cure is obtained.

Itraconazole (400 mg/d) has given promising results in a few patients.

The local application of heat to the lesions may be beneficial.

19   Entomophthoramycoses

19.1   Rhinofacial conidiobolomycosis

19.1.1
Definition

This is a chronic mycosis affecting the subcutaneous tissues. It originates in the nasal sinuses and spreads to the adjacent subcutaneous tissue of the face causing disfigurement.

19.1.2
Geographical distribution

The disease occurs mainly in the tropical rain forests of Africa and South and Central America.

19.1.3
The causal organism and its habitat

Conidiobolus coronatus (Entomophthora coronata) lives as a saprophyte in soil and on decomposing plant matter in moist, warm climates. It can also parasitize certain insects.

The disease is most common among adult males, particularly those living or working in tropical rain forests.

Infection is acquired through inhalation of spores, or their introduction into the nasal cavities by soiled hands.

19.1.4
Clinical manifestations

Conidiobolus infection generally begins with unilateral involvement of the nasal mucosa. The most common nasal symptom is obstruction, but frequent nose-bleeding can occur and is evidence of the development of a nasal polyp in the anterior region of the inferior turbinate. Subcutaneous nodules then develop in the nasal and perinasal regions and may be associated with epidermal lesions.

The spread of the infection is slow but relentless. It is usually confined to the face, and the development of gross facial swelling involving the forehead, periorbital region and upper lip is very distinctive. As a rule, the lesions are firmly attached to the underlying tissue although the bone is spared. The skin remains intact. Spread to the lymph nodes has been reported.

19.1.5
Differential diagnosis

Even if, in advanced cases, the diagnosis is obvious from the appearance, mycological and histological examinations are essential for its confirmation.

**19.1.6
Essential
investigations
and their
interpretation**

MICROSCOPY
Microscopical examination of smears or tissue from the nasal mucosa will reveal broad nonseptate, thin-walled mycelial filaments.

CULTURE
Cultures are far from simple to prepare, and the pathological material must be inoculated on the largest possible number of media; they should be incubated at between 25°C and 35°C.

**19.1.7
Management**

Methods of treatment employed so far have been disappointing. Surgical resection of infected tissue is seldom successful; it may hasten the spread of infection.

The condition can be treated with saturated potassium iodide solution (up to 10 ml three times daily as tolerated) or amphotericin. Long-term results are poor.

19.2

Basidiobolomycosis

**19.2.1
Definition**

This is a chronic subcutaneous infection of the trunk and limbs.

**19.2.2
Geographical
distribution**

The disease is encountered chiefly in the tropical regions in East or West Africa, and South East Asia.

**19.2.3
The causal
organism and
its habitat**

The most widely held view is that *Basidiobolus ranarum* is the sole agent causing the disease, and that *B. meristosporus* and *B. haptosporus* are only synonyms of the former; not all authors are of this opinion, however.

B. ranarum has been recovered from soil and decaying vegetation; it has also been isolated from the gut of frogs, toads and lizards that had apparently swallowed infected insects.

It is still uncertain how the disease is acquired and what is the length of incubation. Inoculation through a thorn prick or an insect bite has been suggested, as has contamination of a wound or other abrasion. The infection is most common in children.

**19.2.4
Clinical
manifestations**

The subcutaneous swelling that characterizes this disease is usually localized to the buttock and thighs, but it may also be found on the arm, leg or shoulder.

The initial swelling may be rapid or slow in onset, and it is hard and painless. The spread is slow but relentless, and a large mass is formed which is attached to the skin but not the underlying tissue (unlike conidiobolus infection). This is a disfiguring infection, but the skin covering the lesions does not ulcerate. Lymphatic obstruction may occur and can result in massive lymphoedema.

There is no functional impairment so long as the joints are not blocked by the volume of the swellings. The underlying bone and joints are not affected by the disease.

19.2.5
Differential
diagnosis

The disease can be diagnosed with confidence on the basis of appearance and the results of the mycological, and particularly the histological, examination.

19.2.6
Essential
investigations
and their
interpretation

Specimens must be taken from the subcutaneous tissue where the infection develops.

MICROSCOPY
Direct microscopy will reveal wide, irregular hyphae or fragments thereof with few septa.

CULTURE
Specimens should be cultured on Sabouraud's agar at 30°C. Identifiable colonies should be obtained in less than 1 week. The colonies formed in culture are wax-like in appearance, finely pleated and grey in colour.

19.2.7
Management

The therapy of choice still appears to be saturated potassium iodide solution (30 mg/kg per day) which should be given for 6–12 months. Oral ketoconazole (400 mg/d) has sometimes been successful, but amphotericin has seldom been helpful. Surgical resection is not curative.

20.1 Definition

The term hyalohyphomycosis is used to refer to infections due to colourless (hyaline) moulds that adopt a septate hyphal form in tissue. This term was introduced in an attempt to stem the proliferation of new disease names each time an organism belonging to a new fungal genus was incriminated as the cause of infection. The number of organisms identified as causal agents of hyalohyphomycosis is increasing, with over 40 different organisms, classified in 17 genera, being listed to date. The term hyalohyphomycosis is reserved as a general name for infections that are caused by unusual hyaline moulds that are not the cause of otherwise-named infections, such as aspergillosis or pseudallescheriosis.

20.2 Fusarium infection

20.2.1 Geographical distribution

These infections are worldwide in distribution.

20.2.2 The causal organisms and their habitat

Members of the genus *Fusarium* are common soil organisms and important plant pathogens. The most frequent cause of human infection is *F. solani*, but *F. oxysporum*, *F. moniliforme* and a number of other species have also been implicated.

20.2.3 Clinical manifestations

Fusarium species have been recognized as one of the most frequent causes of corneal infection (see Chapter 8). In addition, these fungi have been reported to cause infection of nails. Cutaneous infection has been associated with deep skin ulcers, surgical wounds and burns.

Localized deep fusarium infection is rare, but can occur in nonimmunosuppressed individuals. Cases of post-traumatic endophthalmitis, osteomyelitis and arthritis have been reported. Peritonitis has occurred in patients on peritoneal dialysis.

Disseminated fusarium infection is most commonly encountered in neutropenic individuals, particularly patients undergoing intensive antileukaemic treatment and/or bone marrow transplantation. Most infections follow inhalation, but some have followed cutaneous inoculation, such as in cases of catheter-related infection or following toe or finger cellulitis.

The clinical manifestations of disseminated fusarium infection are similar in several respects to those of acute invasive aspergillosis (see Chapter 10). Like the aetiological agents of aspergillosis and mucormycosis, *Fusarium* species have a predilection for vascular invasion, resulting in thrombosis and tissue necrosis. The most common presentation is a neutropenic patient with persistent fever that is unresponsive to broad-spectrum antibacterial treatment. Similar cutaneous lesions occur in both aspergillus and fusarium infection, but are much more common in the latter. These are painful, erythematous, macular or papular lesions that evolve into black necrotic ulcers. These lesions have been noted in about 70% of patients with fusarium infection, compared with less than 5% of patients with aspergillosis.

20.2.4 Essential investigations and their interpretation

Because the tissue form of fusarium cannot be distinguished from that of other agents of hyalohyphomycosis or aspergillosis on microscopic examination, the diagnosis of fusarium infection depends on the isolation of the fungus from clinical specimens, such as blood or material obtained from cutaneous lesions. An important finding has been the high rate of isolation of fusarium from the blood (about 60% of cases), which is in marked contrast to the infrequent isolation of aspergillus and other moulds in similar clinical situations.

20.2.5 Management

The most important factors influencing the outcome of fusarium infection are the underlying condition of the patient and the extent of the infection. Nonimmunosuppressed individuals with localized infection usually respond to treatment.

Patients with fusarium endophthalmitis require surgical debridement and intravitreal instillation of amphotericin. The outcome depends on the extent of the infection. Osteomyelitis will respond to surgical debridement and treatment with parenteral amphotericin. Patients with catheter-related peritonitis have recovered following catheter replacement and amphotericin treatment.

Most patients who have developed disseminated fusarium infection have been neutropenic, and many have died before the disease is suspected. Even with antifungal treatment, the prognosis is poor unless the neutrophil count recovers.

The drug of choice for disseminated fusarium infection is amphotericin. In neutropenic patients, the full dose (at least 1.0 mg/kg per day) must be given from the outset. Provided it is possible, it is prudent to replace central venous catheters.

Amphotericin has been given in combination with other antifungal drugs, but it remains unclear whether the addition of compounds such as flucytosine leads to a more favourable outcome. Itraconazole and fluconazole have been used in too few patients for their usefulness to be assessed.

20.3 Penicillium infection

20.3.1 Geographical distribution

Apart from *Penicillium marneffei* infection, which appears to be restricted in its geographical distribution, these uncommon infections are worldwide in distribution. All natural human infections with *P. marneffei* have occurred in individuals who had resided in or visited parts of East or South East Asia, including southern China, Hong Kong and Thailand.

20.3.2 The causal organisms and their habitat

Members of the genus *Penicillium* are widespread in the environment, being found in soil, dust and decomposing plant matter. Their spores are abundant in the outside air. These ubiquitous moulds are among the most common culture contaminants, but are seldom implicated as the aetiological agents of human infection. The one exception is *P. marneffei*, an usual dimorphic fungus which in lesions appears similar to *Histoplasma capsulatum*. *P. marneffei* has been recovered from bamboo rats in South East Asia and these may provide the natural reservoir for the organism.

In recent years, disseminated *P. marneffei* infection has been reported in European and North American men with HIV infection who had visited South China or Thailand.

20.3.3 Clinical manifestations

P. marneffei infection is often abrupt in onset, with persistent fever, chills, painful cough, weakness and loss of weight being among the common symptoms. Patients often present with generalized lymphadenitis, and hepatosplenic enlargement. Multiple necrotic skin lesions and subcutaneous abscesses are common. Some patients have osteolytic bone lesions and arthritis. The illness is usually fatal if left untreated.

Chest radiographs may reveal localized or patchy infiltrates, abscesses and cavities in the lungs, but the hilar nodes are not calcified.

Human infection with species other than *P. marneffei* is rare. Occasional cases of endocarditis have been reported following valve insertion or replacement. *Penicillium* species have also been isolated from cases of corneal infection and post-traumatic endophthalmitis.

20.3.4 Essential investigations and their interpretation

Because *Penicillium* species are such common culture contaminants, isolation alone is inadequate for making a diagnosis. Even if the same organism is recovered on more than one occasion, the diagnosis remains in doubt unless the fungus is demonstrated in tissue sections. The one exception to this rule is *P. marneffei* which is a well-recognized human pathogen.

Microscopic examination of stained histopathological sections or smears of other clinical material can permit the diagnosis of *P. marneffei* infection if the characteristic elongated cells, often curved and with prominent cross-walls are seen (often within macrophages). *P. marneffei* cells can, however, be confused with those of *Histoplasma capsulatum*.

To confirm the diagnosis, material aspirated from skin, bone or other lesions should be cultured at 25°C and 37°C. Bone marrow and blood cultures are sometimes positive.

20.3.5 Management

P. marneffei infection is a treatable condition, but delay may be fatal.

The drug of choice is amphotericin (1.0 mg/kg per day). The organism appears to be susceptible to flucytosine and some patients have responded to the combination of this drug and amphotericin. Too few patients have been treated with imidazole or triazole drugs for their usefulness to be assessed.

20.4

Other agents of hyalohyphomycosis

Members of the genus *Acremonium* (*Cephalosporium*) are abundant in soil and decomposing vegetation. In humans these moulds have long been recognized as aetiological agents of nail and corneal infections. Occasional deep acremonium infections have been reported in patients with serious underlying medical conditions or other major predisposing factors. Patients with post-traumatic osteomyelitis have recovered following surgical debridement and treatment with amphotericin.

Members of the genus *Paecilomyces* are common in soil.

The two most common species, *P. lilacinus* and *P. variotii*, are common culture contaminants, but these moulds have been implicated as aetiological agents of corneal infection and endophthalmitis. Outbreaks of postsurgical endophthalmitis due to *P. lilacinus* have been reported. Fatal endocarditis has followed valve replacement and sinusitis has also been reported.

The list of other moulds that have been implicated as occasional aetiological agents of human hyalohyphomycosis is lengthening, including members of the genera *Chrysosporium*, *Coprinus*, *Lecythophora*, *Myriodontium* and *Scopulariopsis*.

21   Lobomycosis

Definition

The term lobomycosis (keloidal blastomycosis) is used to refer to a rare, slowly progressive infection of the skin and subcutaneous tissue caused by *Loboa loboi*.

Geographical distribution

Most cases have come from the Amazon region of central Brazil and Surinam. Cases have also been reported from other countries in northern South America and Central America.

The causal organism and its habitat

All attempts to isolate the fungus from lesions of infected individuals have failed. In the dermis it appears as spherical or elliptical budding cells. Although it is accepted that the infection is exogenous in origin, the natural habitat of the causal fungus remains unknown.

The organism gains entry through the skin; it develops *in situ* for an unspecified period (several years) and then reaches the subcutaneous tissue.

The disease is most prevalent in men between 30 and 40 years of age; it is much less common in women and children.

Most infections have occurred in persons who resided in, or travelled frequently through, the tropical forests of Central or South America. Most patients trace their infection to some trauma, such as an insect or snake bite, or cut, or abrasion. There is no human-to-human transmission.

Clinical manifestations

Lobomycosis is an indolent infection which first manifests as a papule or small nodule which is normal skin colour, pink, or with a greyish tinge. The nodule then proliferates and, by partial or total coalescence, may form extensive multilobar lesions. The disease spreads by peripheral extension or autoinoculation due to scratching; or it may follow the draining lymphatics, especially in elderly persons.

The lesions are located in the dermis and subcutis and may form massive tumours, which are at the outset firm and resistant to pressure but later become hard and fibrous, resembling a keloid. If there is ulceration, depressed scars may remain; their surface is smooth and shiny in places owing to atrophy of the underlying epidermis, and wrinkled and fissured in others.

The disease may be symptomless or cause itching and burning; traumas may be especially painful.

The most common sites of infection are the coolest parts of the body; the limbs and face, ears and buttocks. The lesions may cover a whole limb. If the head is involved, the patient may be so grossly disfigured as to be completely excluded from social life.

With a few exceptions there are no adenopathies.

21.5 Differential diagnosis

Lesions of a similar character may be keloid scars or irregular fibrous changes of the skin without secretion. Leprosy, leishmaniasis and chromoblastomycosis can produce similar lesions.

Mycological and histological examination will confirm the diagnosis.

21.6 Essential investigations and their interpretation

21.6.1 Microscopy

Microscopic examination of specimens of pathological material will reveal numerous hyaline, round or oval cells with an average diameter of 9 μm that closely resemble the yeast forms of *Paracoccidioides brasiliensis* or *Histoplasma duboisii*. The cells are enclosed in a double-contoured membrane and are capable of budding. They often form chains and appear to be joined together by bridge-like structures within the chain. If the individual elements show multiple budding, the chains are divided into branches.

21.6.2 Culture

Loboa loboi has never been successfully cultured. This distinguishes it from *Paracoccidioides brasiliensis*, which it closely resembles morphologically.

21.6.3 Histology

The epidermis is irregular in thickness, with parakeratotic zones and sometimes ulcerations and crusts. The dermis underlying it shows hypertrophic and partly hyalinized bundles of connective tissue, between which can be seen granulomatous infiltrates, containing numerous yeasts located extracellularly or phagocytosed by mononuclear and polynuclear cells.

21.7

Management

Antifungal drugs are ineffective. Cure can only be achieved by surgical excision, the extent of the lesions permitting. Unfortunately, however, recurrence after excision is common. In advanced cases, the extensive excision required to remove the lesion may not be justified if the infection is not life-threatening.

The course is slow and chronic and the prognosis poor. Lobomycosis never heals spontaneously nor is it fatal, but it may be a very serious impediment.

22   Mycetoma

22.1   ## Definition

The term mycetoma is used to refer to a chronic suppurative infection of the skin, subcutaneous tissue and bone. It usually affects the hand or foot and may be caused by various fungi (eumycetoma) or actinomycetes (actinomycetoma) which have been inoculated into subcutaneous tissue by minor trauma. A characteristic feature of mycetoma is the production in infected tissue of grains which are compact masses of fungal or actinomycete elements, and their discharge to the outside through sinus tracts.

22.2   ## Geographical distribution

Mycetomas are most common in arid tropical and subtropical regions of Africa and Central America, particularly those bordering the great deserts. However, sporadic cases have been reported from many parts of the world.

The countries surrounding the Saharan and Arabian deserts form the most important endemic area, not only because of the number of new cases occurring each year, but also because of the diversity of causal organisms. Mycetoma is also endemic in certain regions of India and in Central and South America.

22.3   ## The causal organisms and their habitat

Mycetomas are caused by various actinomycetes and fungi that occur as saprophytes in the soil or on vegetation. Individual species of fungi or actinomycetes are often associated with particular geographical areas (see Table 22.1). About six species of fungi are common causes of eumycetoma and five aerobic actinomycetes are common aetiological agents of actinomycetoma. The geographical distribution of these environmental organisms is influenced by climate.

In the arid regions of the tropics and subtropics, the most frequent aetiological agents are *Madurella mycetomatis*, *Actinomadura madurae*, *A. pelletieri* and *Streptomyces somaliensis*. These organisms are encountered in the great Afro-Asian deserts and on their fringes, as well as in southeastern Europe. In the relatively humid mountain regions of Latin America, *Nocardia brasiliensis* is the predominant organism

Table 22.1 Aetiological agents of mycetoma

Species	Geographical distribution	Colour of grain
EUMYCETOMAS		
Leptosphaeria senegalensis	Africa	Black
Madurella grisea	Africa, Central and South America	Black
M. mycetomatis	Worldwide	Black
Neotestudina rosatii	Africa	White
Pseudallescheria boydii	Worldwide	White
Pyrenochaeta romeroi	Africa, South America	Black
Acremonium species	Africa, Middle East	White
Aspergillus nidulans	Africa, Middle East	White
ACTINOMYCETOMAS		
Actinomadura madurae	Worldwide	White/yellow
A. pelletieri	Africa	Red
Nocardia asteroides	Worldwide	White/yellow
N. brasiliensis	Central America	White/yellow
Streptomyces somaliensis	North Africa, Middle East	Yellow/brown

while *M. grisea* is a less prominent cause of infection.

In the occasional cases of mycetoma occurring in temperate regions, the principal isolates have been *Pseudallescheria boydii*, *A. madurae* and *M. mycetomatis*. Other organisms that have occasionally been implicated as causes of mycetoma include *Leptosphaeria senegalensis*, *Neotestudina rosatii*, *Pyrenochaeta romeroi*, *Exophiala jeanselmei*, *Acremonium* species, *Aspergillus nidulans*, *Nocardia asteroides* and *N. caviae*.

Mycetomas occur more frequently in men than in women, adults between 20 and 50 years of age being most commonly affected. However, cases among children have also been reported. Most patients come from rural districts in the tropics and subtropics, although cases often occur in countries with a temperate climate, such as Romania.

Trauma is a critical factor in acquisition of the infection. The organisms may be implanted at the time of injury, or later as a result of secondary contamination of the wound. Traumas are often due to vegetable matter (grasses, wisps of straw, hay). In the tropics and subtropics thorny trees such as the acacia are abundant, and are often used for fuel. Wounds caused by the thorns may facilitate the entry of soil organisms, or the causative agents may grow on the thorns and be implanted directly into the subcutaneous tissue. It is not surprising, therefore, that mycetomas affect mainly the feet of country-dwellers who walk barefoot.

The vast majority of organisms causing mycetomas are saprophytes of the external environment; *Nocardia* species exist in the soil, other species are encountered not only in the soil but also on living and dead plants. However, little is known about their behaviour outside the human host.

22.4

Clinical manifestations

Mycetoma is a chronic, suppurative infection of the subcutaneous tissue and contiguous bones. The lesion appears to begin at a site of minor trauma and continues to spread locally over the ensuing months and years.

The clinical features of the disease are fairly uniform, regardless of the type of organism causing it. Eumycetoma follows a slower and generally less destructive course than actinomycetoma. Spread to the internal organs and involvement of the regional lymph nodes is rare, occurring in no more than 2–5% of cases.

The feet are by far the most common site of involvement and account for two-thirds or more of cases. Other sites include the lower legs, hands, head, neck, chest, shoulder and arms, and the abdomen.

In most cases the first sign of the disease is a small, hard, usually painless subcutaneous nodule which is not attached to the underlying tissue. It is covered by taut thinned skin, which is reddish-violet in colour. A number of small nodules may coalesce to form a larger and frequently multilobar nodule.

Over the ensuing months the nodule begins to soften on the surface, caves in, ulcerates and partly empties, discharging a viscous, purulent fluid containing grains. If there is little fluid, the grains may not escape. The lesion then broadens out at the surface and also spreads inward to infect muscles and bones. The lesions, which are covered with depigmented and scarred skin, present as swellings which are often covered with a crust, but which later develop sinus tracts which discharge pus and blood containing the characteristic grains.

The lesions, which are covered with depigmented and scarred skin, present as areas of softening with ulcerations and sinuses, often covered by a crust.

The infection slowly spreads to adjacent tissue, including bone, often causing considerable deformity. Mycetomas of the feet make the arches convex, thus preventing the toes from touching the ground. However, the general health of the patient is not affected. Pain, burning, and pruritus may occur but are usually mild. Depending on the location and size of the lesion, and also on any bone involvement, limb function may be impaired.

Radiological examination is useful in determining the extent of bone destruction. Abnormalities include periosteal reactions, sclerosis, endosteal reactions, cortical erosions and joint destruction. CT scans are also helpful in delineating the extent of lesions.

Bacterial superinfection is not uncommon and is largely responsible for adenopathies and impairment of the general health. Visceral and especially cerebral metastases are the most serious complications; they cause cachexia and often terminate fatally but are, fortunately, rare.

22.5

Differential diagnosis

In most cases, the diagnosis of mycetoma of the feet presents no problems, but it may be difficult if other body sites are involved, particularly in geographical regions where the disease is not endemic, and if no grains have been discharged at the time of examination.

The characteristic feature of mycetoma is the presence in a fistulated swelling of grains which are found to contain actinomycotic or fungal filaments. This finding distinguishes mycetoma from chromoblastomycosis, cutaneous tuberculosis or from certain syphilitic or leprous lesions, from botryomycosis and other conditions.

22.6

Essential investigations and their interpretation

22.6.1
Gross
examination

The diagnosis of mycetoma depends on the identification of grains. These should, if possible, be obtained by puncture from a softened, but not ulcerated, nodule with a syringe. Failing this, grains can be obtained with a dissecting needle or by aspiration from the secretion flowing from a sinus. If there is no pus flowing from the lesion, small fragments of tissue should be removed. If possible, 20 to 30 grains should be obtained; these should be rinsed in sterile saline before being cultured.

Gross examination of the grains may afford a clue to the aetiological diagnosis (see Table 22.1). Black grains suggest a fungal infection; minute white grains often indicate a nocardia infection; larger white grains the size of a pinhead may be of either fungal or actinomycotic origin. Small, red grains are specific to *Actinomadura pelletieri* but yellowish-white grains may be actinomycotic or fungal in origin. Their shape, consistency and structure must be carefully determined.

22.6.2
Microscopy

Direct microscopic examination will confirm the diagnosis of mycetoma, and also reveals whether the causal organism is a fungus or an actinomycete. Actinomycotic grains contain very fine filaments ($< 1 \, \mu$m diameter) whereas fungal grains contain short hyphae ($2-4 \, \mu$m diameter) which are sometimes swollen. This can be seen by direct microscopic examination of crushed grains in potassium hydroxide, but is much more readily observed in stained histological sections.

22.6.3
Culture

Although the identification of the causal agents of mycetoma can often be deduced from the morphological characteristics of the grains, it is also important to isolate the organism in culture. Agar plates should be inoculated with several grains (or with secretion or tissue fragments) and incubated at $25-30°$C and at $37°$C. The most commonly used agar medium is Sabouraud's agar, without antibiotics but with actidione (cycloheximide) for isolation of actinomycetes, and with antibiotics but without cycloheximide for fungal agents. Alternative media for isolation of actinomycetes include brain–heart infusion or blood agar.

Cultures should be retained for up to 6 weeks before being discarded. The actinomycetes are much slower-growing than the fungi.

22.7

Management

Early actinomycetomas (and some late and advanced cases) respond well to treatment. The drug of choice is streptomycin sulphate (1000 mg/d) given intramuscularly. This should be combined with co-trimoxazole (960 mg twice daily) in cases caused by *S. somaliensis*, *A. pelletieri* and *N. brasiliensis*. Other regimens include co-trimoxazole and amikacin, and streptomycin combined with either dapsone or co-trimoxazole. If no response is seen after 3 weeks of treatment, other regimens can be substituted. These include streptomycin and rifampicin, or streptomycin and sulphadoxine–pyrimethamine. Therapy must be continued for months or even years. In favourable cases, oedema and tenderness regress, discharge of secretion and grains diminishes, and sinuses dry up and close.

It is recommended that, even after symptoms and clinical signs have disappeared, the disease has become clinically silent and laboratory tests have become normal, the treatment should be continued for the same period of time as was required to achieve these results.

The response of eumycetoma to antifungal treatment is disappointing. *M. mycetomatis* and *P. boydii* infection have been known to respond to ketoconazole (400 mg/d), but it is essential to test liver function before starting, and during treatment with this drug. Long-term treatment with itraconazole has resulted in improvement in *M. grisea* mycetoma.

Surgical excision is the method of choice if the eumycotic lesions are small enough for total removal to be possible. Amputation is often required in advanced cases with bone involvement, particularly when there is no response to drug treatment. Prostheses and rehabilitation are indispensable in every case of mutilating surgery.

23   Phaeohyphomycosis

23.1

Definition

The term phaeohyphomycosis is used to refer to subcutaneous and deep-seated infections due to brown-pigmented (dematiaceous) moulds that adopt a septate mycelial form in tissue. This term was also created to segregate various clinical infections due to dematiaceous moulds from the distinct subcutaneous infection known as chromoblastomycosis (see Chapter 18).

23.2

Geographical distribution

Phaeohyphomycosis has a worldwide distribution, but subcutaneous infection is most often seen in the rural population of tropical parts of Central and South America. Most cases of cerebral or paranasal sinus infection have been reported from North America.

23.3

The causal organisms and their habitat

The number of organisms implicated as aetiological agents of phaeohyphomycosis is increasing. More than 80 different moulds, classified in 40 different genera, have been incriminated. Often these fungi have been given different names at different times, and there is therefore a great deal of confusion in the nomenclature used in different reports.

Among the more important aetiological agents can be included *Alternaria* species, *Bipolaris* species, *Curvularia* species, *Exophiala* species, *Exserohilum* species, *Phialophora* species and *Xylohypha bantiana*. Many of these organisms are found in soil or decomposing plant debris; others are plant pathogens. Human infection follows inhalation or traumatic implantation of the fungus.

One common factor among these fungi is their melanin formation in the cell wall in culture and, in most cases, in human tissue.

23.4

Clinical manifestations

Phaeohyphomycosis can be divided into a number of distinct clinical forms, including subcutaneous infection, paranasal sinus infection and cerebral infection.

**23.4.1
Subcutaneous
phaeohypho-
mycosis**

This form of phaeohyphomycosis usually follows the traumatic implantation of the fungus into the subcutaneous
tissue. Minor trauma, such as cuts or wounds due to thorns
or wood splinters, is often sufficient. The principal aetiological agents include *Exophiala jeanselmei, E. spinifera, E.
dermatitidis (Wangiella dermatitidis), Phialophora richardsiae*
and *P. parasitica.*

The lesions occur mainly on the arms and legs. Other less
common sites include the buttocks, neck and face. The
initial lesion is a firm, sometimes tender, subcutaneous
nodule which may enlarge slowly to form a painless cystic
abscess. Lesions are attached to the skin, but not to the
underlying tissue or bone. Unless the cyst ruptures, the
overlying skin remains unaffected.

In immunosuppressed patients with subcutaneous phaeohyphomycosis, the lesions are more likely to drain through
sinuses.

**23.4.2
Paranasal sinus
infection**

This form of phaeohyphomycosis is becoming more common. The principal aetiological agents include *Alternaria*
species, *Bipolaris spicifera, B. hawaiiensis, Curvularia lunata*
and *Exserohilum rostratum.*

It is a slowly progressive condition that may remain confined to the sinuses or spread to contiguous structures.
Affected individuals usually complain of long-standing symptoms of allergic rhinitis, nasal polyps or intermittent sinus
pain. Patients present with nasal obstruction and facial pain,
with or without proptosis. The sinuses are filled with a thick
dark tenacious inspissated mucus.

CT scanning is the best method for evaluating the extent
of the infection. The typical finding is a large mass filling
one or more of the sinuses.

Alternaria and *Curvularia* species have caused necrotic
lesions of the nasal septum in occasional leukaemic and
AIDS patients.

**23.4.3
Cerebral
phaeohypho-
mycosis**

This form of phaeohyphomycosis may follow haematogenous dissemination of infection from the lungs, or it may
result from direct spread from the nasal sinuses. Most cases
are due to *Xylohypha bantiana (Cladosporium trichoides).* Other
aetiological agents include *Bipolaris* species and *Exophiala
dermatitidis.* Many cases of cerebral infection with *X. bantiana*
have occurred in individuals with no obvious factors predisposing them to this condition.

The symptoms of cerebral phaeohyphomycosis are gradual in onset. Persistent headache is the most common presenting symptom. The most frequent clinical findings include focal neurological signs, hemiparesis and fits. Fever is minimal or absent. Chest radiographs are normal.

CT scans of the head will often reveal a unilateral, well-circumscribed lesion, with the frontal lobes of the brain being the most common location.

The CSF findings are varied. The opening pressure may be raised, the protein concentration may be increased, the glucose concentration may be reduced, and pleocytosis may be present. It is most unusual to recover the fungus from the CSF.

The diagnosis is seldom established until neurological resection is performed.

23.4.4
Cutaneous infection

Alternaria species have been seen in, and isolated from, crusted, ulcerated or scaling skin lesions. Many of these infections have followed traumatic implantation and a substantial proportion have occurred in leukaemic patients or transplant recipients. The arms and legs are the commonest sites of infection.

23.4.5
Other forms of phaeohyphomycosis

Dematiaceous moulds have caused endocarditis following valve insertion or replacement and peritonitis in patients on continuous peritoneal dialysis. Post-traumatic osteomyelitis and arthritis have also been reported.

23.5

Differential diagnosis

The lesions of subcutaneous phaeohyphomycosis can be confused with the small initial lesions of chromoblastomycosis, sporotrichosis, blastomycosis, coccidioidomycosis and paracoccidioidomycosis, as well as with cutaneous leishmaniasis. Lymphangitic spread of sporotrichosis and the development of verrucous lesions in the other conditions makes the distinction easier.

In nonimmunosuppressed individuals, the clinical presentation of phaeohyphomycosis of the paranasal sinuses cannot be distinguished from that of aspergillus infection (see Chapter 10). In immunosuppressed patients, aspergillus sinusitis is a fulminant, often lethal, condition unlike phaeohyphomycotic sinusitis. However, both groups of organisms can cause black necrotic lesions of the nasal septum.

Bacterial brain abscess is the most common initial diagnosis in patients with cerebral phaeohyphomycosis. In occasional patients, the diagnosis of cryptococcosis, histoplasmosis, coccidioidomycosis or sporotrichosis must be excluded.

23.6

Essential investigations and their interpretation

Microscopic examination of stained histopathological sections or wet preparations of clinical material, such as pus or skin scrapings, can permit the diagnosis of phaeohyphomycosis if brown-pigmented septate mycelium with occasional branching is seen.

Identification of the aetiological agent is often essential for correct management and this depends on its isolation in culture. Identifiable mycelial colonies can be obtained after incubation at 30°C for 1–3 weeks.

No serological tests are available.

23.7

Management

23.7.1
Subcutaneous phaeohyphomycosis

Incision and drainage of subcutaneous lesions is seldom successful. Surgical resection is required. Treatment with amphotericin has cured or improved nonresectable lesions, but later relapse has been common.

23.7.2
Paranasal sinus infection

Complete surgical debridement combined with amphotericin treatment is essential to halt the progression of this form of phaeohyphomycosis. Even so, it is not uncommon for the condition to recur. The need for repeated debridement is most evident in patients with disabling symptoms or erosion of the bone separating the paranasal sinus from the brain.

Oral treatment with itraconazole (100–400 mg/d) appears promising, although the optimum dosage and duration of treatment has not been defined.

Necrotic nasal septum lesions due to *Alternaria* or *Curvularia* species have been cured following surgical excision.

23.7.3
Cerebral phaeohyphomycosis

In no case has a patient survived without surgical resection of the lesion. Treatment with amphotericin on its own is ineffective. Lesions that have not been completely removed have usually proved fatal.

23.7.4
Cutaneous infection

Surgical debridement of cutaneous lesions combined with parenteral amphotericin is the most effective method of treatment. Topical antifungal treatment is seldom helpful.

23.7.5
Other forms of
phaeohypho-
mycosis

Too few patients have been treated to make firm recommendations. However, the response to amphotericin has been partial at best. Surgical resection of lesions or oral treatment with itraconazole should be considered.

24   Pseudallescheriosis

24.1

Definition

The term pseudallescheriosis is used to refer to infections due to *Pseudallescheria boydii*. This fungus is the most common cause of eumycetoma in temperate regions (see Chapter 22), but it can also cause localized infections of the lungs and other deep organs, as well as widespread disseminated infection.

24.2

Geographical distribution

Mycetoma due to *P. boydii* has been reported from North America. Other forms of *P. boydii* infection have been seen in North and South America, Europe and Asia.

24.3

The causal organism and its habitat

Pseudallescheria boydii (*Petriellidium boydii, Allescheria boydii*) is the perfect form (teleomorph) of the imperfect fungus *Scedosporium* (*Monosporium*) *apiospermum*. *Scedosporium prolificans* (*S. inflatum*) has been isolated from patients with osteomyelitis and arthritis.

P. boydii is a ubiquitous soil-inhabiting fungus. It can often be recovered from polluted water and sewage. Human infection can follow traumatic implantation, inhalation or aspiration of contaminated water.

24.4

Clinical manifestations

P. boydii is the most frequent cause of fungal mycetoma in temperate regions. This chronic infection results from the traumatic implantation of the fungus into subcutaneous tissue (see Chapter 22). The arm and the leg are the commonest sites of infection. The initial lesion is often a small, painless, subcutaneous swelling. This enlarges and ruptures to the surface forming sinus tracts which discharge white grains, then spreads into adjacent tissue and bone, causing disfiguring swelling.

The lung is the second most common site of *P. boydii* infection in humans. In the nonimmunosuppressed person, isolation of the fungus from sputum most often represents transient (or more prolonged) colonization of the bronchi or lungs or both. Underlying cavitating or cystic lung disease is a major factor predisposing an individual to *P. boydii* colonization. Fungus ball formation has been described in patients with residual tuberculous or bronchiectatic cavities. Haemoptysis is a common symptom.

Normal individuals have developed infection of the lung following aspiration of contaminated water; fatal haematogenous dissemination is a frequent complication. In immunosuppressed patients, infection of the lungs often leads to abscess formation or necrotizing pneumonia. Many have developed fatal disseminated pseudallescheriosis.

Localized deep forms of pseudallescheriosis can follow traumatic introduction of the fungus or its dissemination from the lungs. Osteomyelitis, arthritis, sinusitis, endophthalmitis, endocarditis, meningitis and brain abscess have been reported in nonimmunosuppressed individuals. Corneal infection has also been described.

24.5 Essential investigations and their interpretation

The diagnosis of pseudallescheriosis rests on the isolation of the fungus from clinical specimens because the hyaline mycelial form of this mould cannot be distinguished from that of the aetiological agents of aspergillosis or hyalohyphomycosis in smears or histological sections. This distinction is important because the different moulds in these infections differ in their response to antifungal drugs.

The organism has been isolated from CSF specimens in several patients with meningitis, but blood cultures are seldom positive.

24.6 Management

Surgical resection remains the preferred treatment for patients with localized cavitating lesions of the lung. Other forms of pseudallescheriosis, such as sinusitis, arthritis and osteomyelitis, have also been eradicated following surgical debridement of infected tissue. In some cases cure has resulted when debridement has been combined with antifungal treatment.

Most strains of *P. boydii* are resistant to amphotericin, and infections with this fungus are best treated with an azole, such as miconazole, or oral ketoconazole (400–600 mg/d). Itraconazole has proved effective in a few patients.

25   Rhinosporidiosis

Definition
The term rhinosporidiosis is used to refer to a chronic granulomatous infection of the mucous membranes, especially the nasal mucosa, due to *Rhinosporidium seeberi*.

Geographical distribution
Rhinosporidiosis is endemic in India and Sri Lanka as well as in South America and Africa. Occasional cases have been reported from North America, South East Asia and other parts of the world.

The causal organism and its habitat
The aetiological agent is an endosporulating organism, *Rhinosporidium seeberi*. So far, all attempts to isolate this fungus from lesions have failed.

In tissue, large, thick-walled sporangia (spherules) are formed. Large numbers of spores are produced within the sporangia and, when mature, these are released through a pore in the wall. Each spore may develop to form a new sporangium. Little is known about the natural habitat of *R. seeberi*, but it is believed that stagnant pools of water may be the source of human infection.

The disease is most prevalent in rural districts, particularly among persons working or bathing in stagnant water (such as rice fields). Men are more commonly affected than women.

Clinical manifestations
R. seeberi causes the production of large polyps or wart-like lesions that occur predominantly on the mucous membranes. The nasal mucosa is affected in more than 70% of cases.

The onset of the disease in the nose is insidious and the patient remains unaware of its presence until symptoms of obstruction develop. In some cases, the patient complains of itching and unilateral coryza. Rhinoscopic examination will reveal papular or nodular smooth-surfaced lesions that gradually become pedunculated and acquire a papillomatous or proliferative appearance. They are pink, red, or violet in colour. The polyps may obstruct the nasal passages, particularly in the event of even slight trauma. If located low in the nostril, they may protrude and hang onto the upper lips. If they are sited in the posterior part of the fossa, they may partially obstruct the pharynx or larynx and cause dysphagia or dysphonia and dyspnoea.

In some cases the eyes are affected, the lesions being located on the conjuctiva. Initially these are small, flat granulations which may grow in size to form multilobed polyps of a pale pink colour. At the same time there is diffuse vascular dilatation, photophobia, and lacrimation, which is often due to involvement of the lacrimal sac and duct.

The ears may also become involved; depending on their size and location, these polyps may impair hearing.

Lesions may also develop on the male genital organs (penis and in exceptional cases urethra) and on the vulva and vagina in women. They may resemble flat or acuminate condylomas; lesions in the anus present as polyps and may sometimes be mistaken for haemorrhoids.

Cutaneous rhinosporidiosis, which is very rare, is generally due to spread from a neighbouring mucosal lesion. It presents initially as minute papillomas, which gradually become larger and pedunculated. The surface is irregular, verrucous and polypous.

Cutaneous lesions are usually asymptomatic, but because of their location (especially on the sole of the foot) or their size they may cause pain. The surface of ulcerated rhinosporidiosis lesions is dotted with white spots that are more readily discerned when depressed with a glass spatula; on microscopy these are seen to be sporangia.

Dissemination to the internal organs or bones is rare. In most cases the general health of the patient is unimpaired.

25.5 Differential diagnosis

The appearance of pedunculated or unpedunculated polyps or nodules covered with white dots on the nasal mucosa or the conjunctiva should suggest the diagnosis of rhinosporidiosis.

The condition must be distinguished from cryptococcosis, cutaneous tuberculosis, leprous lesions, leishmaniasis and from treponematoses.

25.6 Essential investigations and their interpretation

25.6.1 Microscopy

Microscopy of clinical material reveals round or oval organisms which, depending on age, range in diameter from 6 μm to over 100 μm, with a prominent wall which may be up to 5 μm thick. The sporangia may be filled with endospores.

25.7

Management

The treatment of choice is surgical excision. No drug treatment has proved effective. If left untreated, the polyps will continue to enlarge slowly. In very rare cases, widely disseminated or deep-seated visceral lesions may develop. Spontaneous remission is unusual.

26 Sporotrichosis

Definition

The term sporotrichosis is used to refer to subacute or chronic infections due to the dimorphic fungus, *Sporothrix schenckii*. Following implantation this organism can cause cutaneous or subcutaneous infection which commonly shows lymphatic spread. Occasionally, widespread disseminated infection also occurs.

Geographical distribution

Sporotrichosis is worldwide in distribution, but occurs most frequently in temperate, humid climatic regions. At present, the largest number of reported cases comes from the North American continent. Other regions where the infection is endemic include South America, South Africa and South East Asia.

The causal organism and its habitat

The causative agent is a dimorphic fungus, *Sporothrix schenckii*, which is found in the soil, and on plants and sphagnum moss. It grows in nature as a mycelium, but in tissue it forms small budding cells.

Infection usually follows the traumatic introduction of the fungus into the skin. Minor trauma, such as abrasions or wounds due to thorns or wood splinters, may be sufficient. In occasional cases, infection follows spore inhalation.

It is not clear whether the infection is more common among men than women. Incidence in the different age groups is also variously assessed, but children are less often affected than adults.

Sporotrichosis is most prevalent among individuals who handle soil or plant materials, such as gardeners, florists, mineworkers and carpenters. For this reason sporotrichosis has been regarded as an occupational disease. Sporotrichosis is not transferred from human to human, and the multiple cases that sometimes occur in families or closed communities are usually due to common exposure to the same exogenous source of contamination.

26.4

Clinical manifestations

The clinical manifestations of sporotrichosis are rather variable, which helps to explain the large number of different classification schemes that have been proposed.

The most common clinical presentation is a localized cutaneous or subcutaneous lesion. Lymphatic spread may then lead to the development of further cutaneous lesions. Much less commonly, the fungus may cause infection of the lungs, joints, bones, eyes and meninges. Widespread disseminated infection has been reported in diabetics and alcoholics, in drug abusers and in AIDS patients.

26.4.1
Cutaneous
sporotrichosis

Sporotrichosis tends to affect exposed sites, mainly the limbs and especially the hands and fingers. The right hand is affected more frequently than the left.

The initial lesion develops at the site of implantation of the fungus. It is a painless nodule which is at first movable, but later becomes attached to the neighbouring tissue. The skin turns red, then violaceous, and the nodule breaks down to form an ulcer which discharges a serous or purulent fluid. The edge of the ulcer is often irregular and it may become oedematous, vegetative, and crusted.

After a few days to several weeks the primary lesion may become surrounded by satellite lesions or accompanied by the development of further nodules along the course of the draining lymphatics. These soon become palpable and ulcerate through to the skin. In most cases, however, the lymphangitis heals or remains static for a long time without ulcers forming.

In most cases the regional lymph nodes are not involved. However, this is not an invariable rule. Any involvement of these lymph nodes is evidence of a superimposed bacterial infection and they may ulcerate in turn.

Apart from these very typical lesions, sporotrichosis may present a different clinical picture. Extension over large areas of skin, often described as the disseminated cutaneous form, may occur. Flat, infiltrated or papulopustular or nodulopustular lesions may develop. Whether oozing, proliferative, papillomatous, or verrucous, the lesions of sporotrichosis are generally painless but often pruritic. Several ulcers may be interconnected by subcutaneous fistular passages. Confluent lesions may form a purulent and warty plaque with a continually expanding margin, whereas the centre becomes atrophied, smooth and shiny.

Primary cutaneous lesions may heal spontaneously, leaving behind unsightly and even disfiguring scars, which may be a functional impediment. However, secondary lesions may persist for several years.

**26.4.2
Extracutaneous
sporotrichosis**

Pulmonary sporotrichosis is a rare but well-recognized condition. It may be primary, following the inhalation of spores, and be accompanied by enlargement of the hilar or tracheobronchial lymph nodes. It may, however, also be of a secondary character and due to haematogenous dissemination. The symptoms are nonspecific and include cough, sputum production, fever and weight loss. Haemoptysis may occur and it can be massive and fatal. The course may be chronic. The typical radiological finding is a single, nodular upper lobe lesion, which may or may not cavitate. The natural course of the lung lesion is gradual progression to death.

Most patients with osteoarticular sporotrichosis also have preceding cutaneous lesions. This condition presents as stiffness and pain in a large joint which is indolent in onset. In almost all cases of arthritis, the knee, elbow, ankle or wrist are involved. Osteomyelitis seldom occurs without arthritis; the lesions are usually confined to the long bones near affected joints.

Endophthalmitis, although very rare, may result in blindness; chorioretinitis has also been reported. Cases of meningitis have also been seen.

26.5

Differential diagnosis

The development of a cutaneous lesion on the limbs following trauma is suggestive of sporotrichosis, at least if the patient is resident in an endemic region. The development of multiple ulcers along lymphatics is also suspicious.

At a later stage of development sporotrichosis must be distinguished from mycoses such as blastomycosis, chromoblastomycosis, paracoccidioidomycosis, from leishmaniasis, verrucous tuberculosis and from tertiary syphilis.

The diagnosis ultimately depends on mycological and histological examination.

26.6

Essential investigations and their interpretation

**26.6.1
Microscopy**

Direct examination of clinical material, such as pus or tissue, is often disappointing because the organism is seldom abundant. However, it can be of value if conducted with painstaking care. The detection of typical ovoid-to-cigar-shaped cells or asteroid bodies of *S. schenckii* will confirm the diagnosis.

26.6.2
Culture

The definitive diagnosis of sporotrichosis depends on the isolation of the aetiological agent in culture. Clinical material should be inoculated onto several media, including Sabouraud's agar, and incubated at 22–25°C. Identifiable mycelial colonies will appear in 2–5 days. The colour usually changes from cream or light brown to dark brown or black with age. Confirmation of the identification depends on the morphological characteristics of the mycelial form and its conversion to the yeast form on blood agar at 37°C.

26.6.3
Serological tests

At present, serological tests do not have a significant role in the diagnosis of sporotrichosis. Tube agglutination and latex particle agglutination tests can be used to detect antibodies to *S. schenckii*, but are more helpful in diagnosing the unusual extracutaneous forms of sporotrichosis than in detecting cutaneous infection.

26.7

Management

Saturated potassium iodide solution remains the treatment of choice for patients in developing countries who contract cutaneous sporotrichosis, due to its ease of administration and low cost. The starting dose is 1 ml three times daily, and this is increased to 4–6 ml three times daily. Treatment should be continued for at least a month after clinical cure is obtained, which may take 2–4 months.

If the patient cannot tolerate potassium iodide, oral itraconazole (100–200 mg/d) can be used. Treatment should be continued for up to 6 months. Oral ketoconazole has given poor results.

Local heat, on its own, or used in combination with drug treatment, has been shown to improve cutaneous lesions.

Amphotericin has cured some patients with extracutaneous forms of sporotrichosis, but failures are common. In cases of arthritis or osteomyelitis, better results have been obtained when the drug has been combined with surgical debridement.

Itraconazole (400 mg/d) has given good results in patients with extracutaneous infection.

Introduction

An increasing number of yeasts that had been thought to represent contamination or harmless colonization when isolated from humans have been recognized as significant pathogens in compromised patients. Establishing the diagnosis is difficult and depends on the detection of the organism in histopathological sections or smears of clinical material as well as isolation in culture.

Trichosporonosis

In addition to causing white piedra, a mild superficial infection of the hair most often seen in tropical and subtropical regions (see Chapter 6), *Trichosporon beigelii* causes a localized deep or disseminated infection known as trichosporonosis in immunosuppressed patients. *Trichosporon* species are soil- and water-inhabiting yeasts that are occasionally found associated with human skin, mouth and nails. On the human skin, *T. beigelii* is more frequently found in the genitocrural and perianal regions. The carrier rate of the yeast in the genital region is particularly high in homosexual men.

T. beigelii has been identified as the pathogen in 60 or so reported cases of deep or disseminated trichosporonosis in humans. In each case, the infection developed as a secondary complication of underlying conditions, and most cases have had a fatal outcome.

Disseminated trichosporon infections have mostly been associated with leukaemia, but they have also occurred in patients with multiple myeloma, aplastic anaemia, lymphoma or solid tumours, as well as in organ transplant recipients and AIDS patients. Localized deep infection has occurred in nonimmunosuppressed patients as a complication of cataract extraction, insertion of prosthetic heart valves, intravenous drug abuse, peritoneal dialysis and topical steroid treatment.

Localized deep infection with *T. beigelii* has been described in at least 30 individuals, all of whom had serious underlying medical conditions or other major predisposing factors. *T. beigelii* and a second species, *T. capitatum* (*Blastoschizomyces capitatus*) can cause endophthalmitis, endocarditis and peritonitis in individuals with disrupted anatomical barriers. In recent years, trichosporon infection of the lungs has been reported in leukaemic patients, most of whom had normal neutrophil counts.

Disseminated trichosporonosis is an uncommon but often fatal infection in immunosuppressed individuals. Most cases have occurred in neutropenic patients undergoing anti-leukaemic treatment or bone marrow transplantation. Disseminated infection has also been seen in organ transplant recipients.

The clinical manifestations of disseminated trichosporonosis are similar in certain respects to those of disseminated candidosis (see Chapter 11).

Patients often present with persistent fever that is resistant to antibacterial treatment. Multiple cutaneous lesions occur in both conditions. In patients with trichosporon infection, erythematous maculopapular lesions develop that can progress to disfiguring necrotic ulcers. In neutropenic individuals, trichosporonosis is often fulminant and widespread dissemination can occur. The liver, spleen, lungs and gastrointestinal tract are among the organs most often involved.

**27.2.1
Essential
investigations
and their
interpretation**

The diagnosis of trichosporonosis is seldom suspected until the fungus is isolated from blood, urine or cutaneous lesions. Often, however, patients have died and the infection has remained unrecognized until material obtained post-mortem has been investigated.

MICROSCOPY

Microscopic examination of smears and histopathological sections of cutaneous lesions will reveal branching hyphae with numerous rectangular arthrospores and budding yeast cells. The fungus often grows as small colonies in tissue. When arthrospores are sparse in tissue, *T. beigelii* resembles *Candida albicans*. However, *T. beigelii* sometimes produces more true hyphae and fewer pseudohyphae than *C. albicans*.

CULTURE

In culture, members of the genus *Trichosporon* form either smooth cream-coloured moist or dry heaped colonies that consist of mycelium and pseudomycelium with arthrospores and blastospores. The optimal temperature range is between 29° and 41°C. In neutropenic patients, *T. beigelii* is isolated readily from both blood and skin biopsies. Cultures of bronchoalveolar washes, urine, sputum and faeces have also been positive in neutropenic patients; this finding has not separated colonized from infected patients. *T. beigelii* and *T. capitatum* are distinguished from each other and from other members of the genus on the basis of their sugar assimilation patterns.

SEROLOGICAL TESTS

T. beigelii produces a heat-stable antigen which shares antigenic determinants with the capsular antigen of *Cryptococcus neoformans*. A number of reports have appeared indicating that with serum the latex particle agglutination (LPA) test for *C. neoformans* antigen is postive in patients with disseminated trichosporonosis and could be useful in making the diagnosis. However, negative results have also been obtained in LPA tests with serum and urine specimens from patients dying with disseminated trichosporonosis.

27.2.2
Management

Localized deep trichosporon infection in a nonneutropenic patient will often respond to parenteral treatment with amphotericin (1.0 mg/kg per day). In contrast, in neutropenic individuals, amphotericin treatment is seldom of benefit unless the neutrophil count recovers.

27.3

Malassezia infection

Malassezia furfur (*Pityrosporum orbiculare, P. ovale*) is a lipophilic yeast which forms part of the normal cutaneous flora of humans. It is the aetiological agent of three forms of mild superficial infection: pityriasis versicolor, pityrosporum folliculitis and seborrhoeic dermatitis (see Chapter 6). In recent years it has become apparent that this organism can also cause serious infection in low-birth-weight infants and debilitated adults and children who are receiving parenteral lipid nutrition through indwelling vascular catheters, commonly of the Broviac or Hickman type. Administration of fat emulsions appears to favour the growth of *M. furfur*, leading to colonization of the catheter and subsequent infection. All reported cases have occurred in patients who have received parenteral lipid emulsions through a central venous catheter within 3 days of diagnosis of the infection.

M. furfur catheter-related fungaemia has become a well-recognized complication of total parenteral nutrition (TPN), most cases occurring in infants less than 12 months old. Many of the infants had been born preterm and all required TPN for various underlying illnesses. Due to the severity of underlying illness in many of these patients, it is dificult to assess the precise role of *M. furfur* in clinical status and final outcome of patients.

In infants, *M. furfur* fungaemia seldom remains asymptomatic. Most present with fever and/or apnoea and bradycardia. Interstitial pneumonia and thrombocytopenia are common findings in this patient group. The most commonly reported symptom of systemic infection in infants is fever and respiratory distress with or without apnoea. Other less common symptoms include lethargy, poor feeding, bradycardia and hepatic and splenic enlargement. Of note, no signs of erythema, swelling or purulence have been seen at the entry site of the infected central venous catheter, nor has a skin rash been evident in infants with systemic infection. Chest radiographs have revealed an interstitial, bronchopneumonic or consolidative appearance in 40% of infants.

The few reported adult cases of catheter-associated *M. furfur* sepsis have occurred in conjunction with a variety of underlying illnesses. All patients had been receiving parenteral lipid emulsions through central venous catheters for periods ranging from 3 days to 2 years. Fever was the consistent presenting symptom.

The predominant pathological changes noted in patients with catheter-associated *M. furfur* infections have involved the heart and lungs. These have included mycotic thrombi around the tips of deeply placed catheters, endocardial vegetations and inflammatory lesions of the lung.

27.3.1 Essential investigations and their interpretation

M. furfur fungaemia has sometimes been diagnosed following detection of the organism in stained smears prepared from catheter blood specimens. However, the diagnosis is most often based on isolation of the organism from blood taken through the catheter. The recovery of *M. furfur* from peripheral blood cultures is poor: the number of yeasts isolated is much lower than the number recovered from catheter specimens. Following removal of the catheter, *M. furfur* can often be isolated from the tip.

Although the lipid concentration of conventional broth and agar media is often insufficient to support the growth of *M. furfur*, it would appear that the blood of patients receiving TPN often contains sufficient lipids to permit the initial growth of the organism in culture. Subculture of broth onto an agar medium containing, or overlaid with, a lipid source, should ensure isolation of *M. furfur*. Identifiable colonies can be obtained after incubation for 4–6 days at 32°C.

If *M. furfur* sepsis is suspected, the catheter hub (external connecting port) and tip should be cultured in lipid-containing broth.

**27.3.2
Management**

There are a number of treatment options: discontinue lipids but leave the catheter in place; remove or replace the catheter; give amphotericin without removing the catheter; give amphotericin and remove the catheter.

The most important factor in successful management of this infection is the removal of the infected catheter, whether or not antifungal treatment is given.

Select Bibliography

Comprehensive texts

Kwon-Chung, K.J. and Bennett, J.E. (1992). *Medical Mycology*, 4th edn. Lea & Febiger, Philadelphia. [The latest edition of this authoritative textbook covers all aspects of the diagnosis and management of fungal infections.]

Rippon, J.W. (1988). *Medical Mycology. The Pathogenic Fungi and the Pathogenic Actinomycetes*, 3rd edn. Saunders, Philadelphia. [Another comprehensive textbook which covers all aspects of fungal and actinomycotic infections.]

Monographs on particular aspects

Elewski, B.E. (editor) (1992). *Cutaneous Fungal Infections*. Igaku-Shoin, New York. [This monograph deals with all aspects of superficial fungal infections and also covers the cutaneous manifestations of systemic infections.]

Hay, R.J. (editor) (1989). *Baillière's Clinical Tropical Medicine and Communicable Diseases: Tropical Fungal Infections*. Baillière Tindall, London. [This monograph contains useful reviews of the clinical manifestations, diagnosis and management of many of the fungal diseases encountered in the tropics.]

Roberts, D.T., Evans, E.G.V. and Allen, B.R. (1990). *Fungal Nail Infections*. Gower Medical Publishing, London. [A concise but informative guide to the diagnosis and management of onychomycosis.]

Sarosi, G.A. and Davies, S.F. (editors) (1993). *Fungal Diseases of the Lungs*, 2nd edn. Raven Press, New York. [The latest edition of this comprehensive monograph contains much useful information about pulmonary fungal diseases and their aetiological agents, diagnosis and treatment.]

Smith, J.M.B. (1989). *Opportunistic Mycoses of Man and Animals*. CAB International, Wallingford. [A useful source of information about a number of fungal diseases. Clinical manifestations and management are not covered in detail.]

Vanden Bossche, H., Mackenzie, D.W.R., Cauwenbergh, G., Van Cutsem, J., Drouhet, E. and Dupont, B. (editors) (1990). *Mycoses in AIDS Patients*. Plenum Press, New York. [Individual contributions contain much useful information about AIDS-related fungal infections. Those dealing with the treatment of mycoses in AIDS patients are now becoming outdated.]

Warnock, D.W. and Richardson, M.D. (editors) (1991). *Fungal Infection in the Compromised Patient*, 2nd edn. John Wiley, Chichester. [A recent monograph which contains useful reviews of the clinical manifestations, diagnosis and management of the fungal diseases encountered in AIDS and other groups of immunosuppressed patients.]

Monographs on particular diseases

Bodey, G.P. (editor) (1993). *Candidiasis. Pathogenesis, Diagnosis and Treatment*, 2nd edn. Raven Press, New York. [The new edition of this monograph contains much useful information about the different clinical forms of candidosis and their diagnosis and treatment.]

Odds, F.C. (1988). *Candida and Candidosis*, 2nd edn. Baillière Tindall, London. [This remains the definitive monograph on all aspects of the organisms and the many different forms of the disease.]

Samaranayake, L.P. and MacFarlane, T.W. (editors) (1990). *Oral Candidosis*. Wright, London. [This well-illustrated monograph contains useful reviews of the clinical manifestations, diagnosis and management of the different clinical forms of this disease.]

Stevens, D.A. (editor) (1980). *Coccidioidomycosis*. Plenum Press, New York. [Although the treatment recommendations have become outdated, this monograph remains a most useful source of information about this disease.]

Laboratory diagnosis of fungal infection

Chandler, F.W. and Watts, J.C. (1987). *Pathologic Diagnosis of Fungal Infections*. ASCP Press, Chicago. [The excellent colour photographs and descriptions make this an essential reference text.]

Evans, E.G.V. and Richardson, M.D. (editors) (1989). *Medical Mycology: a Practical Approach*. IRL Press at Oxford University Press, Oxford. [Individual contributions contain much useful practical information about the different aspects of laboratory diagnosis of fungal infection.]

Koneman, E.W. and Roberts, G.D. (1985). *Practical Laboratory Mycology*, 3rd edn. Williams & Wilkins, Baltimore. [This illustrated manual describes the different procedures used for processing and culturing of clinical specimens and the identification of organisms. Serological tests are not covered.]

McGinnis, M.R. (1980). *Laboratory Handbook of Medical Mycology*. Academic Press, New York. [Another manual dealing with procedures for processing of specimens and identification of organisms. The excellent illustrations and descriptions make this an essential reference text.]

Salfelder, K. (1990). *Atlas of Fungal Pathology*. Kluwer Academic Publishers, Dordrecht. [Another well-illustrated manual dealing with the histopathological diagnosis of fungal infections.]

Antifungal chemotherapy

Jacobs, P.H. and Nall, L. (1990). *Antifungal Drug Therapy. A Complete Guide for the Practitioner*. Marcel Dekker, New York. [Most chapters deal with specific infections and the remainder cover particular patient groups, such as children and those with AIDS.]

Ryley, J.F. (editor) (1990). *Chemotherapy of Fungal Disease*. Springer-Verlag, Berlin. [The many excellent contributions to this monograph deal with all aspects of the discovery, development and clinical use of antifungal drugs.]

Introductory texts

Clayton, Y.M. and Midgley, G. (1985). *Medical Mycology*. Pocket Picture Guide. Gower Medical, London. [A short illustrated introduction to the subject with brief descriptions of diagnostic procedures.]

Evans, E.G.V. and Gentles, J.C. (1985). *Essentials of Medical Mycology*. Churchill Livingstone, Edinburgh. [This text is recommended as a clear and concise introduction to the subject. Management of patients is not discussed in detail.]

Kern, M.E. (1985). *Medical Mycology: a Self-instructional Text*. Davis, Philadelphia. [A well-structured introduction to the laboratory identification of fungi.]

Larone, D.H. (1987). *Medically Important Fungi. A Guide to Identification*, 2nd edn. Elsevier, New York. [An illustrated guide to the laboratory identification of fungi.]

Recommended reviews

Bennett, J.E., Hay, R.J. and Peterson, P.K. (editors) (1992). *New Strategies in Fungal Disease*. Churchill Livingstone, Edinburgh.

McGinnis, M.R. (editor) (1985). *Current Topics in Medical Mycology*, Vol. 1. Springer Verlag, New York.

McGinnis, M.R. (editor) (1988). *Current Topics in Medical Mycology*, Vol. 2. Springer Verlag, New York.

McGinnis, M.R. and Borgers, M. (editors) (1989). *Current Topics in Medical Mycology*, Vol. 3. Springer Verlag, New York.

Borgers, M., Hay, R.J. and Rinaldi, M.G. (editors) (1992). *Current Topics in Medical Mycology*, Vol. 4. Springer Verlag, New York.

Index